MASTERING
THE
LIFE
PLAN

Also by Jeffry S. Life, MD, PhD

The Life Plan

MASTERING THE LIFE PLAN

The Essential Steps to Achieving Great Health
and a Leaner, Stronger, and Sexier Body

Jeffry S. Life, MD, PhD

ATRIA BOOKS

New York   London   Toronto   Sydney   New Delhi

ATRIA BOOKS

A Division of Simon & Schuster, Inc.
1230 Avenue of the Americas
New York, NY 10020

This publication contains the opinions and ideas of its author. It is intended to provide helpful and informative material on the subjects addressed in the publication. It is sold with the understanding that the author and publisher are not engaged in rendering medical, health, or any other kind of personal professional services in the book. The reader should consult his or her medical, health, or other competent professional before adopting any of the suggestions in this book or drawing inferences from it.

The author and publisher specifically disclaim all responsibility for any liability, loss, or risk, personal or otherwise, which is incurred as a consequence, directly or indirectly, of the use and application of any of the contents of this book.

First Atria Books hardcover edition March 2013

ATRIA B O O K S and colophon are trademarks of Simon & Schuster, Inc.

For information about special discounts for bulk purchases, please contact Simon & Schuster Special Sales at 1-866-506-1949 or business@simonandschuster.com.

The Simon & Schuster Speakers Bureau can bring authors to your live event. For more information or to book an event, contact the Simon & Schuster Speakers Bureau at 1-866-248-3049 or visit our website at www.simonspeakers.com.

Manufactured in the United States of America

10 9 8 7 6 5 4 3 2 1

Library of Congress Cataloging-in-Publication Data

Life, Jeffry S.
  Mastering the life plan : the essential steps to achieving great health and a leaner, stronger, and sexier body / by Jeffry S. Life, MD, PhD.
     pages cm
  Includes bibliographical references.
  1. Men—Health and hygiene. I. Title.
  RA777.8.L55 2013
  613'.04234—dc23
                                    2012048986
  ISBN 978-1-4516-8170-3
  ISBN 978-1-4516-8171-0 (ebook)

This book, like its predecessor, is dedicated to Alan P. Mintz, M.D.,
"The Father of Age Management Medicine," whose wisdom
and vision set me on the path to find my Life Plan.

Contents

PART THREE

MASTERING THE LIFE PLAN FOR THE REST OF YOUR LIFE 217

MASTERING
THE
LIFE
PLAN

Introduction: Taking Control of Your Health

In the time since my first book came out in 2010 a lot has changed. I went from being a relatively obscure person—known mostly for being "that old guy in those health ads"—to having a national best-selling book, appearing on television and in print magazines, and even being featured coast to coast in the *New York Times* as well as the *Los Angeles Times* in the same week. I'm proud of my program and the scrutiny it has been put under, and I'm even more proud of the thousands of men who have taken the first step toward better health by following it.

Yet at the same time, there are far too many men out there whose overall health has remained unchanged. The vast majority of men are still sitting around watching TV after work, being couch potatoes (or mouse potatoes), and eating poorly and gaining body fat, especially around their bellies. These men still haven't gotten the message that "end of the day fatigue" is not caused by their job, but by their lack of exercise, poor nutrition, and probable hormone deficiencies, putting them at risk not only for compromising their quality of life, but also for disease.

Meanwhile, the economy here and all around the world has tanked, and though we're successfully fighting our way out of a terrible recession, the biggest losers have been men. Simply put, our position in the workplace is plummeting. The majority of people who lost their jobs during the economic downturn were men, and women have been more likely to be rehired.

For the first time in American history the balance of the workforce has tipped toward women. And sadly, many of the men trained for traditional heavy-lifting jobs in construction, factory work, and warehouses are still on the sidelines.

I know just as well as anyone that when you're not feeling well and you've been hit by any kind of psychological blow, whether your house is upside down or you've lost your job, you can't perform as well as you used to in any aspect of your life. These upsets can cause you to fall into a downward spiral of depression and poor health. So it shouldn't be a surprise that the biggest complaint that men have when they come to see me is that they've lost their energy. Yet one thing I have learned is that as men, we can't provide for our families unless we start taking care of ourselves.

In order for men to really succeed in today's tough environment, we have to do better. We need to be high-energy people with a more youthful appearance, and be able to maintain our health and enthusiasm for life as we age. The best way to do this is by staying healthy and fit and lean, and not finding ourselves on the couch, which is a direct path to obesity, poor health, Type 2 diabetes, and heart disease.

The Life Plan is all about recapturing your vital energy and maintaining it as you get older. By mastering my program, you can turn your health around and find that zest for life, whether that means regaining your sexual function or finding your competitive edge in the workplace. You'll find that your renewed energy permeates every aspect of your life, including your relationship with your significant other and relationships with your kids, your grandkids, and your peers.

When you're physically taking care of yourself and you have more energy to do the things that you want to do, and to have the relationships you want to have, it naturally improves your mood and makes you more productive. More energy even makes your thinking better, which is becoming more crucial in today's world. The fact is that the jobs of the future are not physical jobs, they're thinking jobs, many of which women may be intrinsically better at. The bottom line is that taking care of your body is helping you take care of your ability to think, your ability to maintain focus, and your ability to succeed.

What's New?

If this is your first introduction to the Life Plan, then welcome! My philosophy, which I live and breathe, is that it's never too late to reverse disease, improve health, and see lasting change.

I hope that you'll use this book to learn the basics behind the science of my program so that you can begin your own transformation.

Overall, *Mastering the Life Plan* lets you get ready for my program in smaller, simpler steps. In this new book I've outlined exactly what I do every day to stay in great shape. This streamlined version takes much of the Chinese menu approach out of the plan, and instead provides a single, comprehensive diet and exercise program. So if you have been following the program, you can use this book as a way to keep motivated, especially if you are away from home for extended periods of time.

When I wrote *The Life Plan*, my goal was to give men all the information they would need to turn their health around. What surprised me most was how much the media wanted to talk about the concepts of hormone replacement therapies for men. And as each day goes by, I'm still called for my opinion on this aspect of my program, by other doctors, the media, and regular folks just like you. In this book, I'll delve much deeper into the controversy of hormone replacement therapies. You'll have access to the most recent medical studies on the topic, proper dosages, necessary testing, and even more ways to naturally create testosterone, growth hormone, and many of the other necessary hormones on your own. In short, you'll have everything you need to make an informed decision about your health and to have the tools you need to discuss this with your own physician.

This book will also show you how to work the health-care system to make sure that you are getting the care you need. As with any other wellness plan, you'll want to talk to your doctor before you start my program. Let him or her understand that you are interested in a healthy lifestyle that is meant to increase metabolism, prevent disease, and reverse aging. Together, you can join the revolution of healthy aging. Inside this book you'll find a comprehensive list of the medical testing you need at every annual physical, as well as careful instructions on how to get the most out of every doctor visit. This will help you create a wealth of baseline information that you can use to stay vital as you age and limit your exposure to "surprise" illnesses. These "early warning" tests can be used to prevent or delay their onset.

If you've already read *The Life Plan* and enjoyed the success you've achieved on the plan, you'll find that this book makes following the Life Plan even easier. This book includes many more recipes, along with meal plans and shopping lists that any man can manage. Over the past two years I've also discovered how easy it is to get the right nutrition through nutrient-rich shakes. I've created my own line of shakes that have been specifically formulated to fit the dietary needs of men, and recipes for them are included in these pages. Better still, the shakes are so delicious and easy to prepare that you can make them right at home. You'll also learn how to flavor them so that they don't becoming boring. I've also included my best tips and tricks for eating out, especially if you are a frequent traveler. Finally, there is a list of the top supplements you should consider taking, depending on your health and your diet.

I've also streamlined the exercise program so that you can learn how to exercise exactly the way I do. This book features one full resistance training workout that is based on what I do every day. I've focused my new cardiovascular program on spinning. The combination of spinning, my LifeCycle stationary bicycle, and swimming is how I've been getting my aerobic workout in over the past year. The balance/flexibility workout is streamlined so that you can get all three of these types of exercise into your day more easily. For each of these three core areas of fitness, I've also included brand-new workouts for you to do right at home if you don't belong to a gym, or when you're on the road. So there are absolutely no excuses: You can read this book and start exercising today!

How This Book Works

I like to think of this book as a jumpstart to the Life Plan. Once you've mastered the Life Plan, you can move on to the more individualized program that I created in my first book. The book you are reading now is meant to get you up to speed and give you all the tools you need to begin to restore your health.

Part One throws you right into my three-level eating program so you can begin to reverse disease, such as obesity, heart disease, or diabetes, or avoid it entirely. This is not your wife's diet, or your girlfriend's. These diets were created by me, specifically for men, so don't worry: You'll feel satisfied after every meal.

Part Two outlines my unique exercise program, which incorporates every facet of physical fitness, including cardiovascular workouts, resistance training, and balance and stretching exercises based on the Pilates method and martial arts. My Life Plan is different from any other exercise program because it focuses on combining these three core exercise components, what I call the Mighty Three. By doing these types of exercise in combination throughout your week, you will be able to see results quickly, and continue with the program forever. There are dozens of new photographs so that you can follow the directions and watch me complete the exercises, making sure that you are using correct form every time. I've also included a method for you to track your progress for the entire Life Plan.

Part Three gives you everything you need in order to follow the Life Plan for the rest of your life. First, you'll learn about the importance of correcting hormone deficiencies based on the results I've seen in my own life and my medical practice, as well as in peer-reviewed, evidence-based scientific studies. Then, you'll learn how to get the most out of every doctor's visit so that you won't be a hostage to the risk-management model of medicine. Instead, you'll master healthy aging just as if you were in my office.

By following this program, you should start noticing changes in the first two weeks. All it takes is making up your mind to get off the couch. If I can master this type of lifestyle, any man can. So let's take the first steps together, where you can begin to understand not just what you are going to do for the rest of your life, but why.

MASTERING THE LIFE PLAN FOR HEALTHY EATING

CHAPTER 1

The Life Plan Philosophy

As a doctor, I know that the second half of your life can—and should—be the best half of your life. I'm confident saying that even though every day, we are aging. But the truth is, we don't have to feel old. To me, getting "old" means the deterioration of your health accompanied by declining energy levels, loss of sexual function, and loss of your zest for life. I don't want any part of that for myself or my patients, and I bet that you don't, either.

It has now been fifteen years since I began my complete physical transformation. What's so exciting to me is that what I accomplished in just a few months has lasted. Today, not only do I feel great, I've been able to maintain my physique and my good health over all these years. In fact, in many ways, I'm stronger, healthier, and more fit than I was when I first got into shape.

I've been able to stay strong and lean, reduce my cholesterol levels, reduce internal or "silent" inflammation, reduce blood sugar levels, eliminate biomarkers for heart attack and stroke, and avoid diabetes. I have actually stopped the progression of heart disease that, unknown to me, had started when I was in my twenties. I have the mental focus, clarity, and sharpness necessary to keep me more productive and creative than ever. At 74 I'm in love with my wife, working every day building my medical practice, writing best-selling books, training with elite athletes, riding my Harley, playing with my grandkids, and learning more about exercise, nutrition, and preventive medicine. I love my life!

But back in 1998, my future did not look as bright. When I discovered that my own hormone levels were deficient, traditional medicine said that andropause, or declining testosterone, is not a disease but a fact of life, so it shouldn't be treated. When I was losing muscle tissue and strength to sarcopenia, conventional doctors once again said to just accept that I was getting older, and basically, just get over it. But even 15 years ago, I knew that they were wrong. The sad part is, most men continue to hear this same message from their doctors even today.

What most docs still don't get is that aging is not the enemy, and it's not a disease. In fact, by its very definition, aging is a gradual change in your body that doesn't result from disease. Disease is the deviation or interruption of the normal function of any part or system of your body. Each of us has a unique set of inherited predispositions for certain health issues: That's your DNA code. On top of that, your lifestyle choices contribute to whether these tendencies will materialize. Lifestyle can definitely trump genetics. So instead of accepting disease or waiting for it to appear, you can learn how to use my health strategies to keep your body metabolically and physiologically in balance. That's the Life Plan.

The Philosophy Behind the Medicine

I do not accept as fact traditional medicine's proclamation that there's nothing we can do about "natural declines" that occur as we get older, when in fact there's everything we can do about them. When I was on *The Doctors Show* in 2012, the producers cleverly built the segment not only around my book, but around my name. I think the acronym they created really sums up my philosophy (and I wish I'd thought of it myself). This book teaches you how to master these four core areas as we age:

- **L—Levels of hormones:** Reversing hormone deficiencies keeps you energized, vibrant, and healthy. Declining hormone levels are the result of a disease process, not aging, and should be treated. In my opinion it's malpractice for doctors to ignore declining hormone levels and write them off as an acceptable part of aging. Study after study has shown that increasing testosterone and other critical hormone levels in deficient adults greatly affects health in many positive ways, from improving bone mineral density, sexual function, libido, and body composition to reducing risk for heart disease, diabetes, cancer, stroke, and Alzheimer's disease. An optimal level of testosterone can actually decrease or eliminate Metabolic Syndrome, obesity, diabetes, and high blood pressure and cholesterol. And testosterone is not the only hormone you need to be concerned with: Later in the book you'll learn about all of the hormones that you need to be tested for, and how to enhance existing levels if necessary.

- **I—Insulin control:** Maintaining low insulin levels keeps you from getting fat and cascading into poor health, so it's critical to learn how to manage it through diet. Many researchers believe that high levels of insulin cause the other components of Metabolic Syndrome to develop—obesity, high triglycerides, elevated blood pressures, and inflammation. Excess levels of insulin are also thought to be the single most important factor that accelerates the aging process. High insulin levels affect your percent body fat, blood lipid levels, glucose tolerance, aerobic capacity, muscle mass, strength, and immune function. However, when you structure a nutrition program around keeping blood sugars and insulin levels in check as I have, you will get a huge benefit beyond improved health—increased muscle size. In just four to seven days of eating "clean" you can move your blood sugar and insulin levels toward their ideal range, and by two weeks you will no longer be plagued by feelings of hunger, depravation, and cravings. You'll experience a marked improvement in your mental focus, exercise endurance, strength, optimal health, muscularity, and leanness. These are the reasons why my diet plans are all structured to lower insulin levels.

- **F—Food as fuel:** The foods we eat can change our lives by providing constant energy and promoting good health. Your current diet may be filled with processed foods, unhealthy proteins, and sugar-laden simple carbohydrates that all taste great but really accelerate aging. All these bad foods are quickly stored as body fat and arterial plaque. They also suck the energy right out of you, add weight, and create the perfect conditions for stroke, diabetes, heart disease, and Alzheimer's disease. Always remember, what you put into your mouth can either hurt you or help you. I'll teach you how to change the way you eat so that you can begin to lose weight and reverse your potential for illness.

- **E—Exercise:** A comprehensive exercise program can not only transform our bodies, but improve our thinking and even our sex lives with just one hour of working out a day. One goal of the Life Plan is preserving bone density and enhancing muscle tissue growth. Without it, the average American male can expect to gain approximately one pound of body fat every year between ages 30 and 60 and lose about a half pound of muscle mass each year over the same period. At age 60 and onward it gets even worse as the rise in body fat replaces muscle mass. The largest loss of muscle mass occurs between ages 50 and 75, averaging 25 to 30 percent.

The 10 Biggest Myths Surrounding Men's Health

Healthy aging specialists like me are dedicated to the science of healthy aging. We emphasize the enhancement of health over the treatment of illness, focusing on disease prevention, wellness, and quality of life. This approach is based on the fact that today, the majority of men already possess a genetic makeup that will allow us to live well beyond age 85. The key is to make the best of the genes we have so that we can live better, longer. By incorporating these practices into our daily lives we can reverse illness and compress the time we are sick. As I like to tell my patients, we can't stop the aging process, but we can definitely manage it.

Even still, there are many misconceptions that surround men's health, and particularly healthy aging. These myths do nothing but hold men back, and frankly, we need to get rid of them. Another aspect of my philosophy is being completely up to date with the medical literature and backing up all my recommendations with peer-reviewed, evidence-based research studies.

1. *Growth hormone therapy and testosterone therapy are the same as steroid abuse by athletes:* Completely false. Bodybuilders and athletes who use testosterone replacement therapy to enhance their performance are illegally (and dangerously) using hormone therapy in a manner not intended, because they are taking too much and are most probably not deficient. In fact, I'll bet the illegal users aren't getting tested for hormonal deficiencies, but are merely using the drug to ramp up their testosterone levels to as much as 10 to 20 times higher than the upper limits of the healthy range.

   Testosterone replacement therapy needs clinical supervision. Because illegal users' levels aren't monitored via periodic blood work, the concentration of testosterone in their system can reach hazardous levels. However, clinically supervised testosterone replacement therapy for the purpose of counteracting hormone deficiencies and promoting good health is safe and effective, with minimal side effects.

   It's also important to remember that growth hormone and testosterone therapies are prescribed to prevent disease and reverse disease; they will not help you grow muscles and get ripped. I look the way I do because I spend hours at the gym each week working out. This is the most common misconception: that by taking these hormones men can build muscle and get rid of body fat. However, I will say that what hormone replacement therapy has done for me typifies what it has done for my patients. It has helped me create an optimal environment within my body, a healthy environment of hormones that are at healthy levels, which has enabled me to maximize all the training that I do, all the cardio and resistance training and flexibility training, so that I can look like I do at age 74. If I just did all the training and had low hormone levels, I wouldn't look anything like I do now. If I did no training and just took hormones, I wouldn't look anything like I do now.

It is very likely that the same young, professional athletes who are abusing hormone therapies are also working out at elite levels every day. These guys train at such intense levels that to some extent it's questionable whether their athletic performance really benefits from growth hormone or testosterone replacement therapy. I do believe that these therapies make them feel psychologically better and probably allow them to train harder and have fewer injuries. At the same time I know that they are putting themselves at great risk for potentially serious medical problems.

One of the big complaints my patients share with me is that when they start the program, and are going to the gym after not working out for a very long while, it takes them a few days just to recover from just one workout session. Once I correct their hormone deficiencies, that all goes away and they can recover more rapidly, which allows them to work out more often and at a higher level.

2. *Testosterone therapy causes cancer of the prostate and testicles, and other serious health concerns:* Simply wrong! In fact, reversing testosterone deficiencies is one of the key ways to prevent these and other types of cancers. This unfortunate myth has steered the medical community in the wrong direction for 70 years. It started with a 1941 journal article that reported that testosterone injections increased the rate of prostate cancer growth, and that castration decreased it. Yet the problem wasn't with testosterone, it was with the study: It was based on only one patient! Subsequent studies have failed to link elevated testosterone levels with increased risk of prostate cancer. In fact, one large longitudinal study found just the opposite to be true—low testosterone levels were a risk factor for prostate cancer.

Another frequently repeated myth is that testosterone replacement therapy increases the risk for cardiovascular disease. Not so. Again, it's just the opposite. The heart has the highest concentration of testosterone receptors in the body, so testosterone has a huge impact on heart health. Men with healthy testosterone levels have fewer cardiovascular issues and lower mortality rates than those with deficiencies. Other studies link optimal levels of testosterone to reduced risk of coronary artery disease and hypertension, as well as improved cardiac function for those with preexisting heart disease. Older men who undergo testosterone replacement therapy typically see a decrease in LDL and overall cholesterol levels. On the flip side, low testosterone levels have been associated with increased atherosclerosis.

3. *Men don't experience anything like menopause:* While men don't experience a precipitous fall in hormone levels that causes noticeable symptoms as women do, they absolutely do lose hormones as they age, and the results can be just as devastating. The male version of menopause, known as *andropause* or *late-onset hypogonadism,* is not yet universally recognized by the medical community, but its effects are all too real. Men begin to experience a gradual decline in testosterone and other hormones starting in our thirties. By our forties, we may start to feel the effects: decreased libido, erectile dysfunction, decreased bone density, fatigue, weight gain, loss of muscle mass and strength, even anxiety or depression.

   A traditional doctor may shrug off these complaints as the "normal" signs and symptoms of aging and leave it at that. Such medical practices are what perpetuate the myth that andropause isn't real.

   Or they may check your testosterone level and—finding it to be in the "normal" range—allow the problem to go untreated. However, the problem lies in the definition of "normal." The reference range is between 300 and 1,000 nanograms per deciliter (ng/dl). A testosterone "deficiency" is characterized by levels below 200 ng/dl. So if your tested levels are above 200, the traditional physician may think your testosterone levels are fine. The reality is that a low borderline-"normal" test result is equivalent to a D-minus on your report card. Raising your testosterone level to the upper normal range of 700–1,100 is what I look to achieve for my patients, and you shouldn't settle for less either. By reversing hormone loss, you'll reverse the symptoms of andropause and the diseases that accompany it.

4. *Men cannot increase muscle mass and strength as they get older:* Nothing could be further from the truth. I've gained 10 pounds of muscle in the last two years just by doing the right kind of exercise, eating clean, and making sure my hormone levels are at the top end of the normal range. The Life Plan is meant to make sure that we avoid losses of muscle tissue and strength as we age. You'll first learn how to get back into exercise safely so that you can begin to build muscle and get stronger, which will help protect your health for years to come. Then, by following this program, you'll quickly

start to see results as you get leaner and more ripped, which will motivate you to make exercise an integral part of your life.

The truth is that men need to increase muscle mass in order to combat *sarcopenia,* a condition marked by muscle atrophy and loss that typically begins in your thirties and worsens as you age. If you don't exercise properly, muscle loss will progress at the rate of 3 to 5 percent with each decade starting in your thirties and forties, then increase to 10 to 20 percent every decade after that.

5. *Declining sexual function or interest (libido) is a normal part of aging:* If you want to use this as your excuse, go ahead. But I'll show you how to have a vibrant sex life and enjoy every minute of it. Having sex three times a week serves as a key benchmark that you're healthy and physically fit. Yet an estimated 34 percent of all American men age 40 to 70 suffer from some level of erectile dysfunction. Before you fill your Viagra prescription, or talk to your doctor about getting one, there's plenty you can do yourself to get your sex life back on track, beginning with exercise. I'm not talking about using your bed as a trampoline, either. Physically active men over 50 reported better erections—and had a 30 percent lower risk for impotence than their inactive cohorts. Another study of over 40,000 men became the largest study to demonstrate that the more exercise a man does, the less likely he'll experience erectile dysfunction. So once you get with the program, you'll find that your sexual health improves along with your physical health, and you may go back to having the sex life of a 20-year-old.

6. *I'm not a candidate for heart disease because I exercise, my cholesterol is in normal range, and my last stress test was normal:* I wish this one were true, but sadly, it's not always the case. I believe, and the medical literature supports me, that the better care your heart gets—including the right exercise, nutrition, nutraceuticals, and healthy hormone levels—the easier it is to reduce your risk of heart disease. But it doesn't give you a free pass. What's more, over 90 percent of heart attack events in men with significantly diseased blood vessels happen at arterial sites undetectable by conventional diagnostics (that is, stress testing).

Since heart disease is the leading cause of death for men, every strategy in this book is designed to help you prevent or reverse cardiovascular problems. My approach is focused on protecting your endothelium, the thin, one-cell layer lining the interior of the heart and entire vascular tree. The endothelium forms a dynamic interface between your blood and your body. When not properly cared for, your endothelial cells can become dysfunctional and fall prey to numerous disease processes that may cause atherosclerosis, hypertension, inflammatory syndromes, heart disease, stroke, and even dementia. A 2003 Mayo Clinic paper defined endothelial dysfunction as the "ultimate risk" among all the cardiovascular risk factors. So even if you don't have heart disease or a family history of risk, you must still work at improving the health of your endothelium.

7. *Carrying a spare tire is another part of aging that I can't do anything about:* Not true! I used to have a huge belly, and now I'm incredibly lean. Belly fat is hard to get rid of, but not impossible. In fact, belly fat is the last area where you'll see results as you get leaner, but getting rid of it has been a top priority in my life and is a major objective of my Life Plan. That's because it's a pretty clear sign of premature aging and also a huge health risk.

On this program you'll learn how to get rid of the gut with the right exercises and foods you'll actually enjoy eating. For example, a 2011 Harvard study that closely examined weight-loss patterns over 20 years has shown that a diet high in vegetables and whole grains like I prescribe is the best way to lose weight. We also know that certain foods actually increase metabolism and play a significant role in promoting fat loss, including belly fat. The study also found that there are only two foods proven to encourage weight loss: peanut butter and yogurt, both of which you can eat pretty frequently on this plan. On the flip side, the study confirmed what I'm sure you can guess: Every guy's favorite foods—steak, potatoes, sweets, and beer—are literally guaranteed to add inches to your midsection.

I'll show you why a strong cardiovascular exercise program is critical for tapping into belly fat and shrinking your waistline while you shed pounds all over and lower your percent body fat, so that eventually you'll be impressed with your new six-pack.

8. *Retirement is when I finally get to sit back and relax:* If that's your plan, then pick out a new rocking chair and plan to spend plenty of time in it. But that's not what I'm looking forward to. When my dad retired at age 65 he was all about sitting in his La-Z-Boy. That's what his whole generation thought: They were supposed to just stop doing everything. But in reality, the last thing they needed was to sit around and take it easy. By the time my dad was my age he was profoundly deconditioned and had lost much of his muscle mass and strength. Worse, his thinking was cloudy, and he had lost all appreciation for life, to the point that he actually dreaded getting up every morning.

At 74, I'm not at all ready to retire, but when I think about it, I'm hoping that retirement will give me more time to increase my exercise program and do more physical activity outdoors because I'll have more time on my hands. I won't miss workouts because of my hectic schedule. My new condominium has a magnificent indoor two-lane lap pool that's hardly ever used, so I have gotten back into swimming in addition to everything else I do.

If you are new to retirement and out of shape, this is a perfect time to really focus on your own health and well-being. Take advantage of this well-structured program of exercise and nutrition, and use all the tools available to regain your vitality and energy, so that you can really enjoy your retirement and fully participate in whatever is in store for your future.

9. *As you get older you need less sleep:* Not true! As we get older we typically get less sleep because nighttime becomes more interrupted with more intermittent awakenings, but the truth is that you really need the same number of hours of sleep, and maybe even more. During sleep your body repairs itself: It's the time when you produce most of your growth hormone. So sleep is extremely important, and men who are sleep deprived will be the first to tell you that every aspect of their life is affected, from health, to mental clarity, to energy levels, to progression of disease.

If I get less than seven hours of sleep, I'll wake up fine and go to the gym and feel fine until the afternoon, and then I just really start dragging. I start getting aches and pains in my muscles and joints. I also notice that my performance in the gym is not as good: I can't lift as much. But if I get eight hours of sleep, even if I have to get up to use the bathroom, I can go through the day with high energy right up until it's time to go to bed. I never think about taking a nap.

Getting good sleep is vital for better thinking and your overall health. It's also a necessity when it comes to losing weight and keeping it off for good. According to an American Heart Association Conference in 2011, Columbia University researchers have demonstrated that people who get less sleep consume significantly more calories. A good eating and exercise program, like mine, is a key ingredient in increasing your energy, which can then keep you alert and awake throughout the day and help you sleep better at night. You'll also see how an eating plan centered on small, frequent meals throughout the day will provide much more energy than three larger meals.

10. *Memory lapses and brain fog have nothing to do with my overall health:* Not true! Your brain's performance is one of the best indicators of how the rest of your body

is functioning. The brain is a delicate and sensitive organ that requires significant amounts of energy, oxygen, and nutrients. So if you believe that you're not thinking as clearly as you used to, it's not a sign of aging: It's a wakeup call for you to take a good look at your health, and see how you can improve the way your internal systems are working.

Brain fog can include feeling spaced out, forgetful, confused, lost, tired, and having difficulty with concentration. If you're not keeping up in the office or you're slow to remember where you're supposed to be, you may be experiencing the first signs of mild cognitive impairment, or MCI. Luckily, this book will show you how to reverse these symptoms by focusing on the right foods, engaging in smart, frequent exercise, and correcting hormone deficiencies so that you can avoid brain fog, dramatically improve your brain health, and think clearly for years to come.

FEEDBACK FROM MY FANS

NAME: Tyler S.

MESSAGE: I just bought your book at the local Books a Million here in Prattville, AL. I turn 50 in March. All I needed to see was the cover and realize my life is just an excuse. I am taking back control of my health and my desire to live life fully. There is much to do . . . let's get started.

Getting Started

- -

Tyler's right: There's no time like the present to get yourself into better shape. Now that you know where I'm coming from, let's begin by getting your daily eating habits cleaned up. In the next chapter, you'll learn how to master my program for optimal health and determine which of three simple diets you should follow. You can start immediately on any one of these new eating plans, depending on what your weight-loss goal is and your current health status.

CHAPTER 2

The Life Plan Diets

The foods we eat profoundly affect our physical and mental health, our athletic performance, and how we age. Researchers are continuing to uncover the direct links between food choices and the frightening increase in diseases such as diabetes, heart disease, obesity, and more. Yet even with the latest scientific research at my fingertips, making the right food choices has always been the toughest part of my own personal health journey.

The most difficult area in every man's effort to change his body seems to be diet, and my own experience is similar to those of most of my patients. Before my transformation, I ate the wrong foods all the time, and way too much of them—bread and other wheat products, white rice, French fries, ice cream, chocolates, all kinds of sweets, red meat, fried foods, and more than the occasional cocktail. Even today, if I start eating the wrong foods it isn't long before I'm completely off track. So every once in a while, even I need to review the basics of why I have to eat right. Then I take a look at one of my "before" photos, and that's all the motivation I need to get back on the program.

Before I go any further, you need to know that when I talk about weight loss I'm always referring to *body fat loss*. A critical component of my Life Plan is to promote fat loss . . . never muscle loss! In fact, my plan promotes gains in muscle mass, and for good reason: Increased muscle mass makes it easier to burn more calories because it increases your overall metabolic rate.

Most diets focus on weight loss with a total disregard for whether you end up losing fat or muscle. In fact, what typically occurs whenever people follow any other diet for some period of time is that they lose both muscle and fat, and frankly, they're so excited about the results on the scale that they don't really care. Unfortunately, the pattern ends as soon as they start to celebrate their success and slowly go back to their old ways of eating. Before they know it, they've regained the fat lost but haven't restored muscle tissue. That's when people, particularly men, simply become fatter, weaker versions of their old selves. Worst of all, they have lost one of the key components to burning calories—muscle tissue.

If you follow my carefully focused nutrition program, your weight loss will bring lasting positive results to your overall health as your muscle mass increases and your body fat disappears.

Losing Body Fat Improves Your Longevity

There is no greater predictor of premature death than being over-fat. Worse, carrying around more than 10 extra pounds of fat can spell trouble for your thinking now, and later in life. A study in the March 2009 issue of *Archives of Neurology* found that in men, worsening cognitive function correlated with the highest levels of all adiposity measures: The fatter you are, the more likely you will experience cognitive decline later in life. What's more, your weight affects every aspect of how your body functions. Obesity is such an enormous epidemic that we've created a new name for an old problem: Metabolic Syndrome. This occurs when excess weight affects your heart and increases your risk for diabetes. However, Metabolic Syndrome is completely and totally preventable and reversible. Weight loss, exercise, and correcting hormone deficiencies are the keys to preventing this disease as well as losing body fat—especially abdominal fat.

Insulin resistance is the central problem of Metabolic Syndrome. Insulin not only regulates blood sugar, it also plays a very important role in fat metabolism by increasing the secretion of lipoprotein lipase, which increases the uptake of fat from your bloodstream into body cells. The more resistant you are to your insulin, the more insulin your body needs to make in order to maintain your blood sugar levels. And more insulin equals more body fat. So, when insulin levels are kept low, you reduce your risk for all of the serious diseases most Americans die from, you can burn your excess fat for energy, and you are much less likely to convert calories into body fat—a win-win-win situation.

The major cause of insulin resistance is poor nutrition and lack of exercise. It's physiologically impossible for you to burn body fat for energy when insulin levels are high. However, both aerobic and resistance training have been shown to reverse insulin resistance. And as your body fat disappears and your muscle mass increases, your insulin resistance diminishes. You also reduce your need to consume extra calories because your body can now tap into stored body fat more efficiently. This alone is reason why you just can't diet away body fat: You have to burn it off with exercise.

Controlling insulin levels is the primary objective of my nutrition plan. This can best be achieved by eating small meals and carefully controlling your intake of carbohydrates, limiting your choices to those with a low glycemic index (most vegetables and fruits, and a few of the non-wheat whole grains). It is also important to always eat a high-quality, low-fat source of protein any time carbohydrates are consumed. The ratio of protein to carbohydrate needed to achieve ideal insulin control should be between 0.5 and 1.0: This means at least a half portion of protein with every full-size portion of carbs.

A study in the *American Journal of Nutrition* compared diets with the same number of calories but different protein-to-carb ratios. The diet with a protein-to-carbohydrate ratio of 0.6 (similar to my Life Plan Diets) keeps insulin levels low and maintains a positive nitrogen balance. The diet higher in carbohydrates and lower in protein, such as the American Heart Association Diet (with a protein-to-carbohydrate ratio of 0.25), increases insulin secretion and produces a negative nitrogen balance. A negative nitrogen balance means you are breaking down your muscle to provide energy for your body. A positive nitrogen balance, on the other hand, indicates that you are building muscle mass.

As you get more comfortable eating less food, you'll also be reducing the number of free radicals (the unstable atoms that are produced when food is converted to energy) produced when these foods are digested and stored. Many scientists believe that if we can reduce free-radical production in our bodies, we will reduce the damage they do to our cells and dramatically slow the aging process and prevent age-related diseases.

Last, one of the goals of this program is to enable you to increase your own production of hormones, including human growth hormone (hGH). hGH is measured as IGF-1 (Insulin-like Growth Factor-1). As the name implies, Insulin-like Growth Factor-1 is structurally related to insulin. These two hormones share the same receptor sites on cells, creating a competition in which only one hormone will be predominantly effective. A nutrition program that focuses on keeping insulin levels as low as possible will enable you to increase your own natural production of IGF-1. Because you need to optimize growth hormone levels to achieve great health and quality of life, my plan is designed to keep blood sugars low, allowing you to effectively manage your insulin, which will help you achieve healthy levels of growth hormone on your own.

DO YOU HAVE DIFFICULTY LOSING WEIGHT?

Occasionally some of my patients reach a plateau on the program, and they just can't drop any more body fat. This resistance to fat loss can be caused by several factors, including medications. Both over-the-counter (OTC) treatments and prescription medications can affect weight loss. If you are taking any of the following, talk to your doctor to see if there are other alternatives that won't inhibit weight loss. Do not stop taking your medications without speaking with your physician first.

- Antianxiety agents like Lexapro, Cymbalta, Xanax, Effexor, Prozac, Celexa, Valium, Ativan, and Klonopin

- Antiseizure meds like Depakote, Depakene, and Divalproex

- Anti-inflammatories (NSAIDs) from OTCs like aspirin, Advil, and Aleve to prescription meds like Celebrex and Daypro

- Antidepressants like Paxil, Zoloft, Clozaril, Seroquel, Zyprexa, and Risperdal

- Blood pressure medications like Cardura, Inderal, Lotrel, and Caduet

- Diabetic drugs like DiaBeta, Diabinese, and insulin

- Cardiovascular medications like Heparin, Coumadin, and Lovenox

- Antihistamines like Benadryl, Allegra, Zyrtec, and Claritin

- Heartburn inhibitors like Nexium and Prevacid

- Diuretics like Demadex, Aldactone, and Zaroxolyn

- Corticosteroids like prednisone, prednisolone, and cortisone

If medications aren't the problem, make sure you don't have an underactive thyroid gland. The tests listed in Chapter 10 can help you determine if you need to take thyroid hormone replacement medication to correct your resistance to weight loss.

If these aren't the cause of your resistance, then modify your nutrition plan. Begin eating slightly fewer calories. If, after a week, you still haven't broken through, then slowly begin changing your ratio by replacing some of the carbohydrate calories with more healthy fats and protein. It's very likely that if you increase your intake of fat and protein and decrease carbohydrates you will begin seeing better results. And make sure you are doing enough cardio work, which we'll get to later in the book.

Losing Body Fat Increases Your Energy

Metabolism is the energy we expend to maintain all physical and chemical changes in our body. Our metabolic rate reflects how rapidly we use our energy stores. This rate is influenced by many factors, including genetics, natural hormonal activity, body size, and body fat composition. While we can't change our genetics, we can control all the other factors that influence our metabolism. And contrary to popular belief, your age has a minimal effect on your metabolic rate. Instead, it's your hormone levels and level of fitness that are the key components. You also need muscle to keep metabolism high. The more muscle or lean body mass you have, the greater the number of calories you can burn during exercise and subsequently throughout the day.

The foods on the Life Plan are chosen specifically for their ability to increase your metabolism, which naturally increases energy levels. Not only will increasing your metabolism make you feel more alive and awake every day, but you will also be training your body to burn food more efficiently, creating more energy to pump up your workouts and eliminate body fat. This is the good kind of vicious cycle: When you increase your energy, you'll have more energy to exercise, which in turn increases your metabolism to burn more food, leaving you leaner and healthier.

Avoid Sugar at All Costs

I can't say the following often enough: Sugar is toxic, wreaking havoc on your health, and it is a driving force for a myriad of diseases, including diabetes, obesity, hypertension, heart disease, and as the latest research indicates, some forms of cancer. Lewis Cantley, a Harvard professor and the head of the Beth Israel Deaconess Cancer Center, says that when we eat or drink sugar, it causes a sudden spike in insulin, which can serve as a catalyst to fuel certain types of cancers. Nearly a third of some common cancers have insulin receptors on their surface. Insulin binds to these receptors and signals the tumor to start consuming glucose. Many experts are now considering the campaign against sugar as important as the war on tobacco.

By eliminating as much sugar from your diet as possible, you'll be able take more control of your health and stop cravings once and for all, which will help you moderate your appetite. The American Heart Association report recommends that men should not consume more than 150 calories of added sugars a day. That's less than the amount in just one can of soda. However, I know that this is easier said than done. Sugar has become a bigger part of our daily diet than most people realize. Beyond the obvious things such as table sugar, honey, syrup, jams and jellies, sugary drinks, and desserts, sugar can be found in just about every processed food you can imagine, from yogurts and sauces to bread and peanut butter. Unknowingly, Americans now consume 130 pounds of sugar per person a year—that's a third of a pound every day. My advice: Read labels very carefully, and avoid packaged goods that contain sugar or corn syrup. Stop adding sugar to your coffee or sweetening fresh fruit. It's a hard habit to break, but you'll find that in just a week or so you won't feel the urge to reach for the sugar bowl, and you'll find weight loss becomes a whole lot easier.

This is critical to know, because new research is showing that when it comes to sugar, not all calories are created equal. The latest studies from the University of California, Davis suggest calories from added sugars are different from calories from other foods. Researcher Kimber Stanhope found that the subjects in her study who consumed high-fructose corn syrup had increased blood levels of LDL cholesterol and other risk factors for cardiovascular disease, in as little as two weeks of exposure. This study suggests that when a person consumes too much sugar, the liver gets overloaded with fructose and converts some of it into fat, which ends up in the bloodstream and helps generate a dangerous kind of cholesterol called *small dense LDL*. These particles are known to lodge in blood vessels, form plaque, and are associated with heart attacks. Previously, we doctors and scientists believed that these types of plaques were a result of a high-fat diet, and more recently, a high-calorie diet. Instead, it looks like it's the sugar, not the calories, that's the culprit.

YOUR DOCTOR MIGHT NOT KNOW WHAT I DO

In a 2011 article published in *USA Today*, Christy Ferguson, director of the STOP Obesity Alliance, claimed that 78 percent of primary care physicians reported in a survey that they had no prior training on weight-related issues, and 72 percent said no one in their office had weight-loss training.

Rules for Following the Life Plan Diets

I have created three basic rules to help keep you on the right nutrition track:

Rule One: Meal Frequency

Rule Two: Proper Macronutrient Ratios

Rule Three: Plan Your Day

Rule One: Meal Frequency

The only way to lose body fat is to achieve a caloric deficit by decreasing your intake of food and by burning more calories through exercise. Exercise is, by far, the best way to achieve a caloric deficit because it does not trigger the starvation response, it increases metabolic rate, it increases all of the fat-burning enzymes and hormones, it targets body fat rather than muscle tissue for energy sources, and it increases the sensitivity of all cells to insulin so that carbohydrates are burned for energy rather than being stored as body fat.

Scientific studies continue to reinforce the notion that the best way to eat if you want to get rid of body fat, gain muscle, reduce your risks for heart disease and other serious degenerative diseases, and not feel old is to eat five small, balanced meals every day. When your body is presented with too much fuel at any given meal, it will store it as body fat for later use. And, if you continue to take in too many calories at each meal, your body will never learn how to access this stored fuel, and body fat will continue to accumulate in your body.

Instead of eating the traditional three square meals a day, you need to trick your body by eating low-calorie meals (200–300 calories each) every few hours. This constant feeding technique forces your body to process foods as you eat them, using these same calories for energy before they can build up as fat. This technique is the single most important nutritional concept for ultimate leanness and healthy aging: I learned it from bodybuilders who knew this decades before the nutrition and medical world figured it out.

If your body doesn't get the fuel it needs, it will begin the process of *catabolism*: breaking down muscle tissue and converting it into glucose, the body's ultimate fuel, so that it can continue to carry out your bodily functions. Eating small, frequent meals not only prevents catabolism, you will also feel less hungry throughout the day and will need fewer calories at each meal to satisfy your hunger. Best of all, you'll have more energy to perform better during your workouts, and you will drop body fat like never before.

The whole idea of eating more often to lose weight is one of the toughest concepts for me to get across to my patients. I know that it seems counterintuitive that you can lose weight by eating more often. I've got to admit, it took me a long time to really believe it works. But it really does. Once your body gets used to eating every three to four hours you literally become a fat-burning machine. The key is to not give it more calories than it needs at any one time. When I eat one of my small 300-calorie meals, my body literally gets hot and my energy levels increase.

When you eat frequent small meals you also avoid a common problem with most diets—

caloric restriction. When people severely restrict their daily caloric intake their body rapidly goes into a starvation mode. When this happens, your basal metabolic rate begins to slow down. With severe caloric restriction your resting metabolic rate can drop by as much as 40 to 50 percent. Next, you begin metabolizing muscle tissue, converting it into glucose in order to preserve fat stores—that's right, all your hard-earned muscle starts disappearing. And, as if all of this isn't bad enough, the activity of fat-storing enzymes increases and your fat-burning enzymes decrease so that you become very efficient at storing body fat. Your appetite and cravings begin to skyrocket. If you have the willpower to resist these temptations, it won't be very long before lethargy, fatigue, and a total loss of desire to train take over, and your entire program will be sabotaged. The end result is always more fat and less muscle than you had when you started.

There is absolutely nothing that you can do to prevent this from happening except to never allow your caloric intakes to drop below 1,200 to 1,500 calories each day. This will ensure a one- to two-pound weight loss per week, which the American College of Sports Medicine (ACSM) recommends as a safe level for men that ensures mostly fat loss. The more slowly you lose weight the easier it is to hold on to your lean muscle mass and take the fat off. More important, the slower you go, the more likely it will be that you don't put the fat back on.

Rule Two: Proper Macronutrient Ratios

I have a simple rule that will help you balance each one of the five to six meals you'll be eating every day. Each meal's caloric makeup will consist of one-half to one part fat, two parts protein, and three parts healthy carbohydrates.

For example, if you are following the Basic Health Diet, and eating 1,800 calories per day, you'll eat 360 calories per meal for a total of five meals.

1. Fat: 150 to 300 cal/day   or 30 to 60 cal/meal

2. Protein: 600 cal/day   or 120 cal/meal

3. Carbohydrates: 900 cal/day   or 180 cal/meal

Protein and carbs have 4 cal/gram and fat has 9 cal/gram. You can determine the number of grams of each nutrient group you should consume at any meal by dividing the calories per meal by four or nine.

For example: 1 serving of fat: 60 cal/meal/9 = 6.6 grams of fat per meal

CHOOSE HIGH-QUALITY PROTEINS TO BUILD MUSCLE

Protein and its amino acids are the building blocks of muscle, and are an essential part of the human diet for the growth and repair of tissue. Adequate protein is necessary for successfully optimizing hormones, increasing lean body mass, and decreasing body fat. High-quality proteins contain the most amino acids. They include:

- Chicken

- Egg whites

- Fish

- Lean meats

- Low-fat cottage cheese

- Protein shakes

- Soy products

- Turkey

A very convenient, practical, and efficient way to make sure you are getting enough high-quality protein without any added fat or cholesterol is by supplementing your diet with protein-containing nutritionals (e.g., protein powders, meal replacement drinks, sports bars). This is especially important for men who exercise, since an inadequate protein intake is related to the depletion of essential amino acids that occurs during intense training. In addition, high-quality proteins and essential amino acids have a positive influence on our hormonal and immune response to exercise, and they also enhance our ability to adapt to high-intensity training.

The Life Plan Diets all provide about one gram of protein per pound of body weight daily, which falls right into the recommended range for muscle and strength building. You will be eating approximately 30 to 35 grams of protein with each of your small meals. Each serving size of protein is about the size and thickness of your palm, not your entire hand. The palm does not include the fingers or thumb, as some of my patients wish.

THE RIGHT FATS KEEP YOU FEELING SATISFIED

Healthy types of dietary fat allow your body to feel satisfied after eating, build hormones, ensure the integrity of all your cell walls, insulate and protect your organs, and transport nutrients throughout your body. Assessing the many types and forms of dietary fat can seem complicated, but ultimately, the bottom line is: The optimal types of fat are found in natural foods, and the best fats are listed below. Dietary fats found in processed foods are *not* healthy, no matter what the label says. Avoid foods fried in vegetable oils, such as corn and safflower, and eliminate processed foods. For those of you who don't like fish, fish oil supplements are now an option: You should take three to four grams per day. Cooking with olive or canola oil instead of vegetable oil also helps.

Enjoy any of the following in moderation, based on the ratio:

- Bluefish

- Eggs

- Flounder

- Herring

- Lean animal proteins

- Mackerel

- Nuts

- Olives

- Sardines

- Seeds

- Shrimp

- Swordfish

- Wild salmon

THE RIGHT CARBS ENERGIZE YOUR WORKOUTS

Vegetables and most fruits, whether they are fresh, frozen, or even canned, are healthy carbohydrates because they are digested very slowly and their sugars enter our bloodstream in small amounts. Man-made carbohydrates, on the other hand, come from grains that undergo processing that removes most of their natural fiber and nutrients, making them easily digestible and rapidly assimilated by our bodies. These carbohydrates mainline sugar into our bloodstream, pushing blood sugars and insulin levels sky-high. As our blood sugars fall, hunger returns, cravings rapidly follow, and compulsive, uncontrolled eating takes over.

The glycemic index determines how fast a particular food will raise your blood sugar. Diabetics have successfully used the glycemic index for many years to help control their blood sugars. Recently, people who have wanted to lose weight and prevent cravings have used this index. The idea is that when blood sugar and insulin levels are kept low, your body is much less likely to convert sugars to body fat, and food cravings are reduced or even eliminated. This has worked very well for me and my patients. I recommend it to all of you as another tool that can be used to get lean and stay lean.

You can find a glycemic index list of some of the common foods we eat on the Internet at www.diabetesnet.com. Processed carbs generally have very high glycemic indexes (greater than 60), including ice cream, white breads, all white flour products, bagels, white potatoes, bananas, raisins, potato chips, some alcoholic beverages, white rice, and pastas made with white flour.

Low-glycemic-index foods (under 45) include most nontropical fruits and vegetables, regular oatmeal, sugar-free peanut butter, yams, brown rice, sugar-free dairy products, some non-wheat grains, legumes (with the exception of baked beans and Fava beans), new potatoes and nuts.

FOCUS ON THESE FRUITS

Tropical fruits are exactly what you imagine: fruits that grow in hot climates, mostly outside the mainland United States. This list includes pineapple, banana, pomegranate, guava, mango, papaya, and fresh figs, and these are on the "no" list. So are all dried fruits: They are extremely high in sugar because they become concentrated when their water content is removed. Dehydrated or freeze-dried alternatives would be a much better choice.

Here are the best fresh fruit choices that pass the low-glycemic test and that you can enjoy every day:

- Apples
- Apricots
- Berries (any type)
- Grapefruit
- Grapes
- Melons
- Nectarines
- Oranges
- Peaches
- Pears
- Plums

It is absolutely critical that the carbohydrates you eat be mostly those with a low glycemic index to ensure the maintenance of low levels of blood sugar and insulin. Limit your intake of high-glycemic carbs to immediately before and/or immediately after a high-intensity weight-training workout. This will shuttle muscle building nutrients quickly into muscle tissue and promote growth and strength.

HIGH-FIBER FOODS MAKE THE BEST CARB CHOICES

Fiber is vitally important—especially if you want to lose fat without jeopardizing your muscle mass and, at the same time, improve your overall health. On average, American men consume around 10 grams to 12 grams per day, and the recommended intake is 25 grams to 50 grams per day—preferably around 35 grams. In a major study published in the *Journal of the American Heart Association* in October 1999, it was shown that a high intake of fiber reduces not only obesity, but also high blood pressure, other heart disease risk factors, and the probability of many cancers. Some experts even believe fiber plays a greater role in determining heart disease risk than total or saturated fat intake.

Dietary fiber does all this by remaining mostly undigested in your GI tract. This provides bulk to the foods you eat so that undigested food stays in the stomach longer, making you feel fuller and delaying hunger and cravings. Once the food reaches your intestines, it moves along at a faster rate, which slows the release of carbohydrates and fats into your bloodstream, where blood sugar levels remain well controlled and insulin secretion is reduced. Many experts now believe fiber's effect on blood sugar levels is the main reason for its "fat-fighting" properties and other health benefits.

Because fiber makes you feel full, including it in your diet helps you eat much less overall, without even thinking about it. A 2011 study from Penn State proved that people habitually eat about the same *weight* of food every day. In other words, we feel satisfied once the quantity of food we are looking to eat is met, not the total number of calories. So when you eat food that's physically heavier, you'll eat less of it. When you eat high-fiber foods, including vegetables, you consume a higher volume or weight of food with fewer calories—and you won't feel the least bit deprived.

The best fiber sources include whole natural foods such as:

- Beans

- Brown rice and wild rice

- Fruits

- Green, leafy vegetables

- Legumes

- Sweet potatoes

- Ezekiel bread

DRINK WATER, ALL THE TIME

When I had to prepare for the photo shoot for this book, it was imperative that I look my best: I wanted to photograph even better than I did eight years before, which has been featured in numerous print and TV ads. My goal was to sculpt a leaner body (less than 10 percent body fat) with a slightly more muscular physique. What was most surprising to me was that the key factor to my success wasn't only my workouts or hormones, as my detractors would guess. Instead, I was able to meet my goal of slimming down to a new level by drinking lots of water.

Water has long been one of the best aids for weight loss and dieting—but only in recent years has it been getting the recognition it deserves. Even though it contains no nutrients, it works with other molecules in the body to suppress appetite, reduce sodium buildup, and help maintain toned muscles. What's more, water actually helps improve the metabolism of stored fat and turn it into fuel, which helps your liver accelerate its fat-metabolizing speed even further. Drinking water also promotes kidney function, helps you dissolve enzymes/hormones and eliminate waste and toxins (keeping your skin healthy), and, somewhat counterintuitively, stops fluid retention.

When we are properly hydrated our heart and blood vessels work much better, along with all our other bodily functions—we think better, our strength and endurance are better, we feel

PROCESSED FOODS YOU CAN FEEL GOOD ABOUT EATING

- Packaged foods that are minimally processed with the most natural ingredients.

- Peanut butter without any added ingredients: It's a great source of essential fatty acids, while processed peanut butter, and even some "natural" versions, are loaded with sugar and hydrogenated oil.

- Low-fat dairy instead of fat-free: You need some of dairy's good fat, and fat-free products are usually supplemented with sugar to make them tastier.

- Brown rice and natural oatmeal over "instant" varieties: They have lower glycemic indexes.

better, we are healthier, and we will live longer. Without proper hydration, cells cannot pass along any substance that isn't water-soluble. Not surprisingly, degenerative disease and aging begin when you don't get enough water daily. Add poor nutrition to that and you've got the makings of arthritis, gout, clogged arteries, and cancer.

It's also difficult to believe that 70 to 90 percent of your water intake comes from food, yet we still need to drink even more. You don't have to take my word for it. At a 2011 meeting of the American Chemical Society, scientists reported the results of a study that revealed drinking two eight-ounce glasses of water before meals would enable people to consistently lose weight. Subjects who drank water before meals three times per day lost an average of five pounds more than those who didn't up their water intake. The *Journal of Clinical Endocrinology and Metabolism* (*JCEM*) found that drinking water can also increase a body's metabolism, helping burn energy in a process called *thermogenesis*—the calculated energy expenditure that would be required for the water to heat from room temperature to body temperature. According to the study, people who drank 500 ml (two cups) of water increased their metabolic rate by 30 percent, with the increase beginning within the first 10 minutes and reaching its peak after 30 to 40 minutes, and stayed in effect for an average of one hour. This was attributed to thermogenesis. Adequate hydration has the added benefit of helping us eat less by giving us a satisfied feeling.

Your ability to exercise at full capacity is directly dependent on adequate hydration. If you are as little as 1 percent dehydrated (1.5 pounds in a 150-pound person), all body functions suffer, and you will have a 10 percent decrease in your aerobic capacity. To make sure you're adequately hydrated, you should try to drink one-half ounce of fluid per pound of body weight daily. For example, I weigh 185 pounds. That means that I need to drink 92 fluid ounces—11 cups—of water every day. And don't forget to drink between 8 and 16 ounces of water for every hour of exercise you've completed immediately following your workout.

You'll be able to accomplish this by drinking small amounts of water throughout the day. For example, drink one tall glass full before you have your first cup of coffee in the morning and drink 1 to 2 cups of water 30 minutes before you exercise. Drink a half cup (about three large gulps) every 15 minutes during exercise and 1.5 cups to 3 cups over a one- to two-hour period after you finish exercising. When I really focus on dropping body fat and training hard, I carry around a one-gallon jug of water, and I try to consume most of it every day. The best way to tell that you are getting enough fluids is that you should have to make frequent trips to the bathroom, and your urine will be clear, except for when you first go in the morning.

Unfortunately, few beverages work as well as pure water. A few squirts of lemon juice really help make water easier to drink. To mix things up, you can take your water in the form of sparkling water, tea, or coffee. However, the caffeine found in tea and coffee, and even diet sodas, does exactly the opposite of what you want, creating a diuretic effect—meaning it actually results in less water in your body. The same can be said for alcoholic beverages.

I'm also hesitant to recommend increasing your coffee intake because of the caffeine. I know that many people use caffeinated beverages when they are trying to lose weight for the extra energy they provide and their ability to inhibit hunger. But many men are "caffeine sensitive," which means that not only are they adversely affected by caffeine, it can actually act as a food trigger.

Caffeine interferes with *phosphodiesterase*, an enzyme that prevents the overproduction of epinephrine. Epinephrine is the "fight or flight" hormone, causing glucose to be mobilized from the liver and an increased production of glucose from protein reserves (your muscle tissue). It spikes your blood sugar and signals your brain that you aren't hungry. As blood sugars increase, the pancreas is stimulated to secrete insulin in an attempt to bring your blood sugar back to normal. But when too much sugar is removed and blood sugars crash, you'll feel hunger and quite possibly crave sweets to fight off fatigue and irritability. My advice is: If you have trouble controlling eating and are plagued with intermittent cravings for sweets and high-glycemic-index carbs (such as bagels, white bread, and white rice), wean yourself from coffee and see if this helps. My guess is that it will.

My last bit of advice is to can the diet soda. You may think switching a sugary soda option for a diet version is more heart healthy, but research says otherwise. A recent study comparing soda/diet soda consumption with no soda consumption found that subjects who drank diet soda daily had a 61 percent increased risk of stroke, heart attack, or vascular death as compared with those who drank no soda. Even more surprising, the diet soda risk was almost 50 percent greater than the risk of the regular soda. The upshot: Stay away from both—drink water!

Rule Three: Plan Your Day

As soon as you wake up in the morning, think through where you are going to be eating, and how you will be able to access the food you need for five to six healthy meals. This might mean preparing meals in advance and taking them with you so that you don't find yourself hungry and trapped, pulling into a fast-food restaurant and eating a high-calorie, high-fat, low-nutrition meal.

Here are some of my best planning tips:

1. Cook enough protein and veggies to have meals ready in the fridge or freezer for several days. This is a huge time-saver! Also, check out my website (www.drlife.com) for my new Meal Plan that ensures you will always have the right kinds of food available every day.

2. Always pack lunches and snacks to take with you wherever you go, especially when you are flying. You'll not only save money at restaurants, but you won't eat foods that you know are bad for you when you are on the road and feeling hungry. Even one fast-food hamburger can ruin your motivation for a whole day, or more.

3. Keep meal replacement bars or shakes in your desk drawer to combat midday hunger.

4. Plan according to your day's activities—you can eat bigger, higher-carb meals before a workout, and smaller meals in the evening when you are winding down.

5. Always carry water with you—a no-calorie way to fill yourself up between meals.

6. Don't go to parties or out for dinner when you are hungry. Drink a large glass of water and eat a piece of fruit before you leave so that you'll have more control later.

7. When eating out, tell the server not to bring bread to your table. In fact, stay away from bread and wheat products as much as possible.

8. Use your Food Journal (see Chapter 8) daily. And make a copy of it to keep at work so that you can fill it in when you are in the moment of eating, instead of trying to remember what you ate at the end of the day.

9. Plan your day so that you are not spending too much time near your kitchen or pantry. Don't make this diet harder on yourself by hanging out in the kitchen.

10. Clean out your fridge and pantry and place the foods you'll be eating daily toward the front.

11. Throw away anything that you won't be eating: You're never going back to it. You can donate unopened boxes or cans to local food pantries.

12. Have a small meal before you do your weekly food shopping. Shop the perimeter of the store; that's where the freshest and healthiest foods are located.

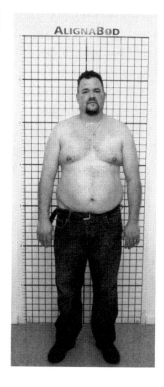

When I was 42 I had a heart attack. Even though I was never in great physical shape, it really took me by surprise. I was six-foot-one, 260 pounds, and I was very lethargic, unmotivated, and tired all the time. I guess you could say that food was my life. I'm a chef at one of the large casinos in Las Vegas. I work in the banquet department, so I do a lot of weddings and corporate functions: very rich, extravagant, high-end food, so I'm surrounded by good food all the time, and a big part of my job is tasting what we prepare before it is served. But I wasn't just tasting: I'd be taking a few extra bites if it was real good (and it almost always was), and that was on top of all the meals I was eating during an 8- to 10-hour shift. At the end of my shift, I was too tired to start cooking for my family. Instead I would just stop and grab some fast food for dinner.

Then one day I was home with my family, and the next thing I knew I was in the hospital. It happened so fast. Right then I promised myself that if I could make it back home I would start all over and take care of myself for once.

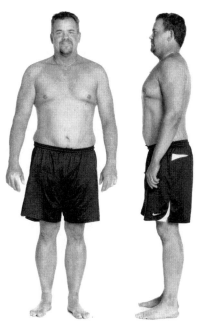

I'd seen Dr. Life's billboards in town, but I also knew his personal trainer, Rod Stanley, who is a friend of mine. His wife and my wife knew each other growing up. Rod had been bugging me to come and train with him for about six months before I had the heart attack. He actually offered to train me for free because I was a friend, but he told me that I had to be dedicated and willing to work, and I knew at that time I wasn't, so I didn't want to waste his time. I told him straight up that I wasn't ready. That was a mistake. Now I'm ready.

I've been working with Dr. Life for about three weeks, and already I can see a huge change in my appearance. I'm already down to 248 and I haven't felt this good in years. After the heart attack I thought I had started eating better. I did eat a lot more salad and stuff but I would still splurge and have a cheeseburger and this and that. Dr. Life explained how I needed to eat clean and live clean all the time. Now, before I eat something, I think about my body more and what changes I really want to create. That makes it easier for me to make the right decisions, not only for me, but for the rest of my family. After my first meeting with Dr. Life, I sat down with the whole family and told them that his program was going to be a lifestyle change for all of us. Now I'm not bringing home fast food. I'm going to the store and buying fresh for them. I have to bring them along slower than I'm doing it, but I'm trying to change the whole family's diet.

Dr. Life and Rod put me on a workout schedule that I can manage. I actually meet him at the gym in the morning. We do a full-body resistance training workout three times a week: Monday, Wednesday, and Friday. I do cardio plus stretching or Pilates every day.

I know the program is working because I feel great and have lots of energy. I'm still on my feet and working long hours, but at the end of the day I feel tired but not physically, more mentally. I'm also taking what I've learned and I'm applying it at work. One of the areas I'm involved with is the employee dining room. We're now adding to the options what we call a "Jim's Plate," named after the president and CEO of MGM Corporation, Jim Marin. He's also trying to get everybody to eat healthier. We've created six new recipes that are a full meal containing 700 calories or less. A lot of the employees are looking at me and the results I've gotten and they are getting motivated, too. What I'm noticing is that in the employee dining room, where we serve all the food for free, and there's a large variety to choose from—cheeseburgers, cheesecakes, all that—people are starting to eat the Jim's Plate because they're seeing results. And guess what we're serving on the Jim's Plate? The same foods that Dr. Life recommends. So, not only am I doing right for myself, now I'm helping other people.

My goal weight is 210, but Dr. Life doesn't want me to focus on that: He thinks that my focus should be about being healthy. Hopefully this program will reverse my heart issues: Dr. Life said as long as I follow his plan it should make an enormous difference. He believes that if I can get my weight under control and get my body leaner then I won't have to take the medication for the rest of my life. With my diet changing and the exercise, he thinks I can reverse most of my problems. I know that I'm very new at this, but I can see my path. I'm just happy to have this opportunity. His last name says it all, Dr. Life. I feel like he's given me my life back.

The Life Plan Shopping List

It's best to start any diet with a full pantry. That will take the guesswork out of what you are going to eat, and where you are going to find it. Below is a list of all the foods I used to create the three meal plans and all the recipes in Chapter 3. If you are going to follow the plan exactly as I recommend, you will need all the following. If you want to go off script, you can swap some of these out only for the good suggestions mentioned above. It's important to remember that any of these whole food items (fruits, veggies, proteins) are acceptable snacks, just make sure to parcel them out in no more than 300-calorie portions. You'll also notice that most of the items on the list are fresh, unless otherwise noted. That's because I know that most men are short on time, and these frozen or canned versions are real time-savers. However, if you want to substitute fresh for canned, all the better.

- Almonds
- Apples
- Asparagus
- Blueberries
- Broccoli
- Brown rice
- Cabbage
- Canned black beans
- Canned chicken
- Canned green beans
- Canned tuna (packed in water)
- Carrots
- Cashews
- Cauliflower

- Celery
- Cherries
- Chicken breast (boneless and skinless)
- Chicken broth (reduced sodium)
- Cottage cheese, low-fat
- Cucumbers
- Distilled white vinegar
- Eggs
- Ezekiel 4:9 sprouted grain bread
- Ezekiel 7 whole grain pocket bread
- Ezekiel 4:9 sprouted grain cereal
- Garlic
- Grapefruit
- Grapes

- Greek yogurt, low-fat
- Hummus
- Iceberg lettuce
- Kale
- Lemon
- Mushrooms, white
- Mustard
- Natural reduced-fat peanut butter
- Nonfat cooking spray
- Olive oil
- Olive oil mayonnaise
- Onions
- Oranges
- Organic tempeh
- Pork loin (lean, boneless)
- Quinoa
- Red bell peppers
- Rolled oats
- Salmon (fresh)

- Seitan wheat protein
- Shrimp
- Smoked salmon
- Soy sauce, low-sodium
- Spinach
- Stir-fry vegetables (fresh or frozen)
- Strawberries
- String cheese, low-fat
- Sweet potatoes (yams)
- T-bone steak (all visible fats removed)
- Tofu, low-fat, extra firm
- Tomatoes
- Turkey breast (boneless, skinless)
- Turkey breast lunchmeat (nitrate/nitrite free)
- Turkey jerky
- Vegan sausage links, low-sodium
- Whey protein
- Whipped cream cheese, low-fat
- Wild rice

WHY I LOVE EZEKIEL BREAD

First, I just like saying the name, which was inspired by the Holy Scripture verse Ezekiel 4:9: "Take also unto thee Wheat, and Barley, and beans, and lentils, and millet, and Spelt, and put them in one vessel, and make bread of it." It turns out that when you actually bake these grains together, you create a bread that doubles as a complete protein that closely parallels the protein found in milk and eggs. In fact, the protein quality is 84.3 percent as efficient as the highest recognized source of protein, and it's made from all vegetable sources. This bread is also rich in vitamins, minerals, and natural fiber, without added fat.

I did a quick experiment to confirm the bread's low blood sugar impact. I checked my blood sugars every 15 minutes for one hour after eating. There was no increase in my blood sugar, and I am very carbohydrate sensitive.

Best of all, it actually tastes good. Try it served warm to release its exceptionally rich, nutty flavor. However, don't look for it in the bread aisle: It's often kept in the refrigerated cases of health food stores and most supermarkets. This is the only type of bread that you should be eating.

The Life Plan Diets

I have devised three simple nutritional plans that create a stepped dieting approach toward the ultimate goal of completely clean eating. Each of the diets is low glycemic, designed to reduce blood pressure and cardiovascular disease while improving overall health and body composition. They focus on natural foods that you can find in any supermarket.

Depending on your current health and fitness level, you can enter into any one of these plans at any point, and upgrade from one to the next. Obviously, the more limiting diets will achieve the best and fastest results.

Everyone should start with the Basic Health Diet and stick with it for at least a week. Rotate through the three days of suggestions at least twice. If you enjoy the diet, you can stay on this level forever. When you are following the Basic Health Diet, you will be having five meals a day at three- to four-hour intervals. The recipes and menu suggestions for these healthy food choices can be easily prepared by steaming, grilling, or stir-frying with small amounts of oil. Follow this rotation for the next three days and then repeat. You can also mix up the days, but try to keep the meals together. In the next chapter, there are simple recipes that you can substitute in as well if you prefer to cook your meals once a week, as I do. There are also more recipes and meal suggestions in *The Life Plan*.

If you are currently a vegetarian, go straight to the Heart Health Diet. However, many vegetarians are dangerously low in energy-creating nutrients, protein, essential amino acids, iron, vitamin B12, calcium, vitamin D, and zinc. The risk of these nutritional deficiencies is even greater while you are following an intense muscle- and strength-building program, like the one you will be following in this plan. Because of this, I strongly recommend that vegetarians take great care in planning, selecting, and preparing nutritious meals to make sure they are getting adequate amounts of essential nutrients. Not only is it important to include the essential micronutrients (vitamins and minerals) and macronutrients (carbohydrates, fats, and proteins) in your nutritional plan, it is also helpful if each meal consists of one portion of carbohydrate and one portion of protein. A portion of each is about the size of a clenched fist or the palm of your hand. If you attempt to boost your protein content for a meal by mixing two high-carbohydrate, moderate-protein sources (such as beans and rice), you will be eating more than one portion of carbohydrate and less than one portion of protein. This can result in fluctuating blood sugar levels and elevates insulin secretion, which can increase fat storage, decrease fat burning, and heighten hunger cravings. My Heart Health Diet helps prevent much of this.

Once you are ready, move to the next level: the Fat-Burning Diet. The Fat-Burning Diet is more rigorous, but it is absolutely the best way I know to get rid of body fat. As with Basic Health, you can stay on this diet forever.

If you still want to increase your weight loss or if you have already been diagnosed with a heart condition, have a stent, or had bypass surgery, high blood pressure, or other vascular problems, move to the final level: Heart Health. Your goal should be to follow the Heart Health Diet as closely as possible forever. This is a completely vegan diet that combines low-glycemic eating with a low-fat diet so that you can start reversing blood vessel disease. Moreover, if you are having problems with your sexual health, this is the diet to follow.

Follow this eating plan carefully. It is very important that you never skip a meal and that you eat five small meals, each having around 300 calories, daily. Make sure that you consume most of your calories before 6 p.m. Eating like this sends signals to your body that you are not starving even though you are creating a caloric deficit, which normally makes you store fat. You are actually tricking your body and making it a fat-burning machine.

The Basic Health Diet

Food	Cal	Fat	Pro	Carb
BREAKFAST 1 (mix ingredients together and cook as instructed on package)				
½ cup rolled oats	190	32	3.5	7
2 oz blueberries	84	0.4	1.1	21.5
3 egg whites	51	0.2	10.8	0.7
BREAKFAST 2				
1 cup low-fat cottage cheese	81	1.1	14	3.1
1 cup strawberries	46	0.4	1	11.1
1 oz raw unsalted almonds	164	14.3	6	5.6
BREAKFAST 3				
4 oz smoked salmon	133	4.9	20.7	0
1 tbs low-fat whipped cream cheese	23	1.8	1.1	0.7
1 slice Ezekiel bread	80	0.5	4	15
1 cup grapes	62	0.4	15.6	0.6
SNACK 1				
3 oz turkey jerky	203	2	38.5	2
1 large 7.9 oz apple	116	0.4	0.6	30.8
SNACK 1				
4 oz canned tuna (in water)	131	0.9	28.8	0
1 stick low-fat string cheese	80	5	8	0.5
2 oz celery	8	0.1	0.4	1.9
SNACK 1				
3 hard-boiled eggs, 2 yolks removed	112	5.4	13.5	1.1
1 large 6.5 oz orange	86	0.2	1.7	21.7

Food	Cal	Fat	Pro	Carb
LUNCH 1				
4 oz turkey breast meat (nitrate/nitrite free)	118	1.9	19.4	4.8
1 Ezekiel 7 whole grain pocket bread	90	0.5	3	19
1 oz tomato	5	0.1	0.2	1.1
4 oz 2-leaf iceberg lettuce	1	0.1	0.1	0.3
1.5 tsp olive oil mayo	50	5	0	0
Place ingredients into pocket bread				
LUNCH 2				
4 oz grilled chicken breast	186	4.1	35.1	0
1 large 7.9 oz apple	116	0.4	0.6	30.8
1 oz almonds	164	14.3	6	5.6
LUNCH 3				
1 cup brown rice	216	1.8	5	44.9
4 oz broiled shrimp	112	1.2	23.7	0
8 asparagus spears	26	0.2	0.2	2.8
SNACK 2				
1 scoop whey protein shake (prepare as directed)	110	0.75	22	0.5
4 oz cherries	71	0.2	1.2	18.1
1 oz cashews	157	12.4	8.6	5.2
SNACK 2				
8 oz low-fat Greek yogurt	173	4.7	22.7	9.3
½ cup blueberries (mixed with yogurt)	42	0.2	0.5	10.7
SNACK 2—PREPARE A SANDWICH				
4 oz canned chicken	120	2	26	0
2 slices Ezekiel bread	160	1	8	30
1.5 tsp olive oil mayo	50	5	0	0

Food	Cal	Fat	Pro	Carb
DINNER 1				
4 oz T-bone steak	200	8.4	29.4	0
1.5 cup steamed kale	50	0.7	3.3	10
6 oz yam	197	0.2	2.5	46.9
DINNER 2				
5 oz broiled salmon	292	17.6	31.3	0
1 cup steamed broccoli	55	0.6	3.7	11.2
1 cup wild rice	83	0.25	3.25	17.45
DINNER 3				
4 oz lean boneless broiled pork loin	237	11.1	32	0
1 slice Ezekiel bread	80	0.5	4	15
4 oz grilled asparagus	26	2.9	2.9	4.9

The Basic Fat-Burning Diet

This low-glycemic diet excludes red meat and dairy fat (such as cheese and milk). Just beyond the Basic Health Diet, this plan removes the biggest sources of saturated/plaque-building fat, which plugs your arteries. Eliminating this source will actually stop the progression of plaque—and in some cases, reverse plaque buildup. The combination of low-glycemic eating while consuming less than 10 percent of your calories from fat sets you on a heart-healthy path.

When I'm not extensively training, I follow this diet. When you are following the Fat-Burning Diet, you will be having five meals a day at three- to four-hour intervals. The recipes and menu suggestions for these healthy food choices can be easily prepared by steaming, grilling, or stir-frying with small amounts of oil. Follow this rotation for three days and then repeat. You can also mix up the days, but try to keep the meals together. In the next chapter, there are simple recipes that you can substitute in as well if you prefer to cook your meals once a week, as I do. There are also more recipes and meal suggestions in *The Life Plan*.

GUESSTIMATING CALORIC VALUES

Use the food charts in this chapter to help you determine the caloric value of typical servings of lean proteins, fruits, and vegetables. Each one of your five meals should be 300 calories or less.

Food	Cal	Fat	Pro	Carb
BREAKFAST 1				
½ cup rolled oats, cooked	190	32	3.5	7
2 oz blueberries (mix with rolled oats)	84	0.4	1.1	21.5
3 oz low-fat tofu	90	2	12	6
BREAKFAST 2				
1 scoop whey protein shake (prepare as directed)	220	1.5	44	1
1 cup strawberries	46	0.4	1	11.1
1 oz raw unsalted almonds	164	14.3	6	5.6
BREAKFAST 3—EGG WHITE OMELET				
6 egg whites	102	0.4	21.6	1.4
1.5 tsp olive oil for cooking	50	5	0	0
1 cup spinach	7	0.1	0.9	1.1
¼ cup tomato	7	0.1	0.3	1.5
1 cup grapes	62	0.4	15.6	0.6
SNACK 1				
3 oz turkey jerky	203	2	38.5	2
1 cup cucumber slices	14	0.2	0.7	2.6
2 oz hummus	94	5.4	4.5	8.1
SNACK 1				
4 oz canned tuna (in water)	131	0.9	28.8	0
1.5 tsp olive oil mayo	50	5	0	0
1 cup (8.2 oz) fresh strawberries	74	0.7	17.9	0.6
SNACK 1				
1 scoop whey protein shake (prepare as directed)	110	0.75	22	0.5
7 to 9 oz large apple	116	0.4	0.6	30.8

Food	Cal	Fat	Pro	Carb
LUNCH 1				
4 oz turkey breast meat (nitrate/nitrite free)	118	1.9	19.4	4.8
1 Ezekiel 7 whole grain pocket bread	90	0.5	3	19
1 oz tomato	5	0.1	0.2	1.1
4 oz–2 leaf iceberg lettuce	1	0.1	0.1	0.3
1.5 tsp olive oil mayo	50	5	0	0

Place ingredients into pocket bread

Food	Cal	Fat	Pro	Carb
LUNCH 2				
1 cup canned black beans, heated	227	0.9	15.2	40.8
4 oz roasted turkey breast	158	1.4	34.1	0
LUNCH 3				
1 cup brown rice	216	1.8	5	44.9
4 oz broiled shrimp	112	1.2	23.7	0
8 asparagus spears	26	0.2	0.2	2.8

Food	Cal	Fat	Pro	Carb
SNACK 2				
1 scoop whey protein shake (mix water/almond milk)	110	0.75	22	0.5
4 oz cherries	71	0.2	1.2	18.1
1 oz cashews	157	12.4	8.6	5.2
SNACK 2				
4 oz hummus	188	10.9	9	16.2
2 oz carrots	20	0.1	0.4	4.6
2 oz celery	8	0.1	0.4	1.9

Food	Cal	Fat	Pro	Carb
SNACK 2—PREPARE A SANDWICH				
4 oz canned chicken	120	2	26	0
2 slices Ezekiel bread	160	1	8	30
1.5 tsp olive oil mayo	50	5	0	0

Food	Cal	Fat	Pro	Carb
DINNER 1				
4 oz roasted chicken breast	187	4.1	35.2	0
1.5 cup steamed cabbage	50	0.9	2.3	10.1
½ cup quinoa, cooked	111	2	4	20
DINNER 2				
5 oz broiled salmon	292	17.6	31.3	0
1 cup steamed broccoli	55	0.6	3.7	11.2
1 cup wild rice	83	0.25	3.25	17.45
DINNER 3				
5 oz shrimp, cooked	140	1.6	29.6	0
1 cup stir-fry vegetables	50	2	2	9
¾ cup brown rice	162	1.3	3.8	33.6

The Basic Heart Health Diet

This is my most extreme approach: a low-glycemic, vegetarian diet. The only good fats allowed are fish oil capsules. Poultry, fish, and nuts are best left out of this diet, but I have included a few for those who just can't live without them. Do your best to minimize these.

This diet is definitely not for the first-time dieter, but it yields great results. This is a research-based plan that is perfect for men with known heart disease—those who have had angioplasty, stents, bypasses, or high coronary calcium scores. Significant research has shown that following this type of diet can reverse plaque and vascular disease. This purely vegetarian approach (with less than 10 percent fat) is the only diet shown to reverse heart disease. Research has demonstrated that vegetarians had not only more optimized cardiac function, but also improved vascular reactivity, lower blood pressure, balanced blood sugar levels, good cholesterol scores, and trimmer bodies.

If you are already following a vegan diet, the best way to make sure you get enough quality protein on this diet is to eat a variety of plant foods that have complementary amino acids. This can best be accomplished by eating a mixture of grains and legumes (rice and beans)—these contain all the essential amino acids that your body needs. Tofu is also an excellent source of high-quality plant protein because it contains all the essential amino acids and has an added bonus of phytochemicals that protect you against heart disease and cancer. In addition, don't forget that nuts are an excellent source of protein, although they are high in fat.

When you are following the Heart Health Diet, you will be having five meals a day at three- to four-hour intervals. The recipes and menu suggestions for these healthy food choices can be easily prepared by steaming, grilling, or stir-frying with small amounts of oil. In the next chapter, there are simple recipes that you can substitute in as well if you prefer to cook your meals once a week, as I do. There are also more recipes and meal suggestions in *The Life Plan*.

Food	Cal	Fat	Pro	Carb
BREAKFAST 1				
3 oz low-fat tofu (pan fry ingredients with a nonfat cooking spray)	91	2	12.1	6.1
1 oz onion	12	0.1	0.3	2.9
1 oz red peppers	41	3.6	0.3	1.9
½ small grapefruit on the side	64	0.2	1.3	16.2
BREAKFAST 2				
1 scoop whey protein shake (prepare as directed)	220	1.5	44	1
1 tbs natural reduced-fat peanut butter	95	6	4	6
1 large 7 to 9 oz apple	116	0.4	0.6	30.8
BREAKFAST 3				
½ cup rolled oats, cooked	152	2.7	6.6	25.9
2.4 oz blueberries	39	0.2	0.5	9.9
4 hard-boiled eggs, yolks removed	68	0.4	14.4	0.8
SNACK 1				
1 cup cucumbers	14	0.2	0.7	2.6
4 oz hummus	188	10.9	9	16.2

Dip cucumbers into hummus

Food	Cal	Fat	Pro	Carb
SNACK 2				
4 oz canned tuna (in water)	131	0.9	28.8	0
1.5 tsp olive oil mayo (mix with tuna)	50	5	0	0
1 cup (8.2 oz) fresh strawberries	74	0.7	17.9	0.6
SNACK 3				
½ cup canned beans	147	0.2	8.6	28.5
7 to 9 oz large apple	116	0.4	0.6	30.8
1 tbs. natural reduced-fat peanut butter	95	6	4	6
LUNCH 1				
4 oz flax tempeh	220	9	20	16
1 Ezekiel 7 whole grain pocket bread	90	0.5	3	19
1 oz tomato	5	0.1	0.2	1.1
4 oz–2 leaf iceberg lettuce	1	0.1	0.1	0.3
Place all ingredients inside pocket bread				
LUNCH 2				
1 cup canned black beans, heated	227	0.9	15.2	40.8
1 cup boiled kale	36	0.5	2.5	7.3
LUNCH 3				
1 cup brown rice, cooked	216	1.8	5	44.9
4 oz broiled shrimp	112	1.2	23.7	0
8 asparagus spears	26	0.2	0.2	2.8
SNACK 2				
1 scoop whey protein shake (prepare as directed)	110	0.75	22	0.5
4 oz cherries	71	0.2	1.2	18.1
1 oz cashews	157	12.4	8.6	5.2

Food	Cal	Fat	Pro	Carb
SNACK 2				
4 oz canned chicken	120	2	26	0
2 oz carrots	20	0.1	0.4	4.6
2 oz celery	8	0.1	0.4	1.9
SNACK 2				
1 large apple	116	0.4	0.6	30.8
1 tbsp natural reduced-fat peanut butter	95	6	4	6
DINNER 1				
1 cup black beans, heated	227	0.9	15.2	40.8
1.5 cup steamed cabbage	50	0.9	2.3	10.1
1.5 cup cauliflower	38	0.2	3	8
DINNER 2				
4 oz tempeh	260	6	22	30
1 cup steamed broccoli	55	0.6	3.7	11.2
1 cup reduced-sodium chicken broth	17	0	3.3	1
DINNER 3				
5 oz reduced-fat tofu	152	3.4	20.3	10.1
1 tbsp olive oil for cooking	120	14	0	0
1 cup stir-fry vegetables				

Keep Reading for More Choices

- -

The next chapter includes more tips and tricks for mastering the Life Plan Diets, including delicious and easy recipes that you can swap into these diets to give you more control and more choice during the program.

ASK DR. LIFE

NAME: Tom C.

QUESTION: Some time ago, I saw about the last fifteen seconds of an interview with Dr. Life. It was on the Fox Network. I heard enough to look for his book. When I found it, I went right into it. I found that he began his journey to health at about the same age I'm at now, which was encouraging. There is a problem, though: food selection. I have real physical problems with foods like beans, peas, cottage cheese, etc. What can I do to get on the Life Plan without consuming foods that affect me adversely?

ANSWER: Tom, you're not the only guy who can't tolerate foods like beans and cottage cheese. On the Life Plan, there are many foods to choose from, so I would listen to what your gut is telling you and avoid the ones that cause problems or discomfort. There are no "secret" foods that will make all the difference on the program: These suggestions are all equally effective in helping you lose body fat and keeping it off for good. So eat what you enjoy from these lists, and focus on how your body responds. You may have to stick with the basic program, which offers more choices, even if it means that it takes you longer to get optimal results compared to others who can move right into the Heart Health or Fat-Burning Diets.

CHAPTER 3

My Favorite Foods

I'm not going to lie: Dieting can be difficult. But there are ways that you can make it easier for yourself so that you don't fall back into your old eating habits. For me, a big part of what keeps me going is my mind-set. I look at eating as just another part of my workout: It's what I know I have to do for my body in order to look good and feel great. That's why the diets listed in Chapter 2 are so rigid. I know that if I follow them exactly, I will be able to maintain my weight.

But the truth is, I can be that limited for only so long. Every couple of weeks, when I can't take those meals any longer, I start to experiment. I don't go off script: I know I have to stay within the context of the original shopping list. I just mix up the ingredients and come up with something new. The recipes that follow are some of my best efforts. I typically swap one of these into the rotation weekly. I also use the recipes in *The Life Plan*.

Sometimes, all it takes is spicing up my meals. I can easily add or swap one type of spice for another to create a completely different taste experience. I love spices because they are completely calorie-free and, when I use them liberally, contain tons of important nutrients. My favorites, and the ones I head to first, are the fresh herbs, such as chopped dill, cilantro, and basil. When I can't get to the store to buy fresh, I use the dried varieties of herbs and include some spices as well: Curry seasoning, anise, red pepper flakes, and cinnamon are my go-to choices.

Lastly, if you have absolutely no desire to set one foot in the kitchen, I've come up with another way for you to follow the Life Plan Diets. I have partnered with a new meal delivery program called Personal Trainer Food. This service is perfect for those who want minimal hassle and ultimate simplicity for meal planning. Now you can get great-tasting, simple-to-prepare,

COUPLES BENEFIT FROM WEIGHT LOSS

Some guys are simply blessed, especially if they have a spouse or partner who will do all their cooking for them. If this is the case, you will likely reap many benefits from this diet that go far beyond your weight loss. Studies have proven that couples who diet together see better results. In fact, couples who lose weight together are also more likely to keep the weight off. According to a 2010 Israeli study of spousal dieting, the *wives* of men who were participating in a weight-loss program lost weight themselves—even though they weren't officially dieting. And we also know that women who feel better about their body image enjoy sex more and are interested in having it more frequently. According to a study from 2000 published in the *International Journal of Eating Disorders*, women who are more satisfied with body image reported more sexual activity, orgasm, initiating sex, greater comfort undressing in front of their partner, having sex with the lights on, trying new sexual behavior, and pleasing their partner sexually than those who have a negative body image.

extremely affordable, and conveniently planned meals that follow the Fat Burning Diet cooked and delivered right to your door via FedEx. All of the meals are pre-cooked, frozen, individually bagged "real" food . . . not TV dinners. Check it out on my website (www.drlife .com). We call it the Life30-Day Meal Plan. It may be just right for you.

The Science Behind My Favorite Foods

If you are the chef in the household, or if you are predominantly cooking for yourself, think of the kitchen as a science lab, and you won't feel less manly about spending lots of time there. As you've learned, there is a distinct science behind eating healthfully, and that doesn't just end with the shopping list. The way you prepare your foods significantly affects their nutrient levels.

Vegetables are able to achieve higher antioxidant levels when they are heated. But in most cases, boiling them will strip away their valuable nutrients. It's best to avoid cooking vegetables with water that is later discarded. If your vegetables are cooked in stews and soups, then the nutrients are retained, so that's a different story. The best way to maximize their nutrient content is by using a microwave, pressure cooker, or steamer.

Animal proteins should always be thoroughly cooked. On the Basic and Fat-Burning Diets, you can still have lean proteins like fish and poultry. The best ways to cook these are without additional fats in order to keep the calorie count down and keep them uncontaminated with bad fats. When you do need to cook with fats, use the right oils, such as olive or canola oils that are rich in omega-3 fatty acids, and stay away from butter and margarine. Broiling and grilling are the cleanest, best-tasting options that require the least amount of additional fats for the cooking process. Microwaving can be fat-free but often leaves proteins feeling rubbery, so it's not my first choice. Baking and sautéing typically require a sauce to keep fish or poultry moist, which makes for poor options as well.

When it comes to cooking grains, I like to use microwave brown rice that comes in individual packets instead of steaming a whole pot. That also allows me to forgo the chicken broth that I used to use for extra flavor: Instead, I season the cooked rice with a little sea salt and fresh ground pepper, which is a much healthier alternative.

The following are some of my favorite foods, and why they are important to include in any of the meal plans:

Almonds: high in healthy fats along with vitamin E, vitamin B, niacin, and riboflavin.

Blueberries: a super food if there ever was one. These antioxidant-rich berries prevent inflammation, promote better thinking, and are one of the most powerful antioxidants.

Broccoli: this nutrient-rich veggie helps stimulate the immune system and protect against damage. It contains vitamins A and C, a healthy amount of fiber, plus glutathione and sulforaphane (anticancer agents).

Cabbage: contains glutathione—a "tripeptide" that prevents cellular damage caused by free radicals.

Eggs: considered to be a perfect protein, but their yolks have gotten a bad rap over the last several years, and this is because they have fairly high levels of saturated fat and cholesterol, which are thought to contribute to heart disease. However, egg yolks can be an excellent source of omega-3 fatty acids. In order to get the most benefit, look for eggs that are marked as "high in omega-3s".

Grapefruit: packed with vitamin C and flavonoids to support your immune system. They also have far fewer calories than oranges or orange juice.

Low-fat yogurt: yogurt's live/active cultures help you battle colds by activating your immune system, and as I mentioned in Chapter 1, it's on the very short list of foods that actually increase metabolism. Try higher-protein Greek yogurt since it's creamier and triple-strained to remove the whey.

Mushrooms: excellent choice to boost your immune response. Mushrooms of all varieties are rich in the mineral selenium, as well as B vitamins (riboflavin and niacin).

Natural peanut butter: one of my very favorite snacks because it's an excellent protein source. Read labels very carefully and choose one that has absolutely nothing added besides roasted peanuts. Along with yogurt, it's one of the few foods that will keep you feeling satisfied and help you burn calories.

Red bell peppers: loaded with vitamin C (double other vitamin C–rich veggies/fruits) and beta carotenes, which give the red-orange pigment, protect cells from free-radical damage, and enhance immune system function.

Spices: spices contain phytonutrients and tons of antioxidants. The following are used in the recipes below, but purchase the ones you like and work with those: basil, dill, parsley, thyme, turmeric, and cayenne pepper.

Spinach: truly a "superimmunity" food, spinach helps new cell production, DNA repair, and strengthens your body's immune system because it is high in the B vitamin folate, as well as vitamin C and fiber.

Sweet potato: another beta carotene–rich food, sweet potatoes are high in fiber and are a great source of vitamin A, which your skins needs to look younger and protect your immune system. Substitute a yam every time you have a hankering for a potato.

Become a Bag Man

My wife, Annie, has great ideas for recipes, but she doesn't have a lot of time to cook. So when I started my transformation 15 years ago, we realized quickly that we had to figure out a way to prepare the foods I needed to eat in order to make dieting effortless for me. For us, that meant cooking large batches of meals every once in a while and then freezing them so I could pop out a serving whenever I wanted.

This has become a huge time-saver for me, and one of the best ways that I've been able to master the Life Plan. If you follow our lead and become a Bag Man yourself, then you will never be more than a freezer away from healthy food. I keep some at home and take several to work with me and keep them frozen until I'm ready to eat them.

Now, when it's time to eat, I can quickly microwave a completely balanced meal: one bag of protein, one bag of a low-glycemic carb (yam, wild rice, or brown rice), and a serving of healthy vegetables. I simply make a small cut into each of the bags, just enough to release steam. I then microwave for two to three minutes, depending on the density of the contents. Then I let it stand for one minute in the bag before I eat so that it can finish cooking and cool down.

Every Bag Man needs a food vacuum sealer, which wraps what you've cooked in plastic and keeps it airtight. These sealers are very simple to operate, and the results are significantly better than traditional zipper bags, foil, plastic wrap, and containers, even if you try to make them airtight. Choose a model that uses a plastic that is BPA-free so that dangerous chemicals are not added to your food during cooking.

I follow one of Annie's recipes below, or the ones I have in *The Life Plan*, doubling or tripling the batches instead of making just one serving. After each meal is finished, I let it cool. Then, I seal individual portions with the vacuum sealer, mark the outside of the packets so that I remember what they are, and then freeze.

Another thing I often do is grill or broil a tray full of boneless, skinless chicken breasts or fish fillets and vary the spices on every five servings. I sprinkle some of them with dill, and then cover them with lemon or orange slices; others are curried, chili-flavored, Tuscan Italian–flavored, or whatever I want, depending on the spice mixes I have on hand. This way I make an entire month's worth of protein choices in one sitting and don't have to face the same flavors night after night.

I do the same with my veggies. I create individual steamer servings instead of cooking at every meal. I quickly parboil the veggies just until they darken in color, no more than two minutes. Then I season with herbs, let dry, and freeze. When it's time to heat them, just microwave for a minute less than if they were fresh, so that the reheating process doesn't overcook them. You can also buy frozen individual servings of vegetables at the grocery store.

Go Easy on Salt

Most of us really don't have to worry about how much salt we eat. About 20 percent of men are salt-sensitive, and when these people consume salt they retain excess fluid. This extra fluid leads to an increase in circulatory volume, which, in turn, increases the work the heart must perform and can also increase blood pressure.

However, you do need to watch your sodium-potassium ratio. Keeping your heart healthy also requires that you consume more potassium. A recent national study found that a sodium-to-potassium ratio under 1 has a protective effect on cardiovascular disease. The easiest way to get more potassium and less sodium is by eating more fruits/vegetables and fewer processed foods. A typical doughnut: 210 mg sodium and 120 mg potassium. A cup of strawberries: 2 mg sodium and 233 mg potassium. And even though you may have heard that bananas are high in potassium, they're still on the "no" list because they are very high in sugar.

If you are not salt-sensitive and don't have a family history of hypertension (high blood pressure), you can continue to use salt in cooking in moderation. I recommend sea salt because it's a coarser grind, which will get you in the habit of using less. Once you cut down on salt you will begin to appreciate other flavors in foods and become less inclined to crave processed foods or fast foods that are typically loaded with the white stuff.

THE EASIEST WAY TO MAKE RICE

The easiest way I've found to prepare rice is with a rice cooker. I use 2½ cups of a blend of long grain brown rice and wild rice with 2 cups of nonfat low-sodium chicken broth (or vegetable broth) and 3 cups of water. Then I turn the machine on and set the mode to "rice cooking" and wait until it's done—usually about 40 minutes.

This makes enough rice for an entire week of meals. I freeze it in single-serving (½ to 1 cup) containers. When I want to have rice, I simply microwave the serving until heated through (approximately 4 minutes if frozen or 2 minutes if thawed).

Mastering the Recipes

Almost all of Annie's recipes are very simple and can be used on any of the diets. The following notations indicate the diet plan that applies to each: Basic Health Diet (BHD); Fat Burning Diet (FBD); and Heart Health Diet (HHD). All of the lunch and dinner recipes can be doubled or tripled if you want to prepare food ahead of time. I suggest that you go fresh for breakfast. This shouldn't be a problem, because these suggestions really don't involve much cooking.

Breakfast

HIGH-POWERED OATMEAL (BHD, FBD, HHD)

Serves 1

½ cup steel cut oats

2 cups water

2 scoops whey protein powder (40 g)

½ cup fresh blueberries

In a 2-quart saucepan, bring water to boil. Stir in oats, cover, and reduce heat to low. Simmer slowly and stir often until oats are desired thickness (approx. 15 minutes). Remove from heat. Stir in protein powder and berries and serve.

YOGURT BREAKFAST CRUNCH (BHD, FBD, HHD)

Serves 1

1 cup Greek low-fat yogurt

½ cup Ezekiel 4:9 sprouted grain cereal

½ cup blueberries or strawberries

Combine all three ingredients into one bowl and serve immediately.

VEGAN BREAKFAST SKILLET (BHD, FBD, HHD)

Serves 2: This is a perfect breakfast for two, but if you are eating by yourself, save half for tomorrow or for a snack later in the day. This dish can be refrigerated and eaten at room temperature.

½ tbs olive oil

¼ medium onion, chopped

½ red bell pepper, chopped

3 oz vegan sausage links, cut into ¼-inch slices

½ pound extra-firm tofu, drained, pressed, and cut into ½-inch dice

6 oz spinach, stemmed and chopped

1 clove garlic, minced

Juice of ½ lemon

½ tsp dried basil

½ tsp dried parsley

½ tsp dried thyme

¼ tsp turmeric

½ tsp salt

Pinch ground cayenne

Heat olive oil in a large skillet over medium-high heat. Add the onion and cook for 2 minutes.

Add the red pepper and veggie sausage links and cook 2 minutes, or until the pepper starts to soften and the sausage begins to brown. Add the tofu, spinach, and garlic. Cook, stirring, for 5 minutes, or until the tofu begins to turn golden. Add the lemon juice, herbs, salt, and cayenne. Cook for 10 minutes to allow the flavors to blend. If the mixture is dry, add a splash of water.

COTTAGE CHEESE AND FRUIT SALAD (BHD, FBD, HHD)

Serves 1

1 cup low-fat cottage cheese

1 cup mixed fruit: choose your favorites from the shopping list

Mix together and enjoy.

POACHED EGG WITH SMOKED SALMON (BHD, FBD)

Serves 1

I like to make these eggs for breakfast and lunch when I want a hot meal. They are perfect for the Life Plan because they do not require any added fat for cooking, and they make a great alternative for when you are sick of hard-boiled eggs. Tip: The poaching pot is much easier to clean if it's still warm from cooking.

1 large egg

Distilled white vinegar

⅛ lb smoked salmon

Cucumber slices (optional)

Break the egg into a small bowl. Fill a large, deep saucepan with at least 3 inches of water. Add 1 tsp of vinegar per cup of water in the saucepan. Bring to a boil. Reduce to a gentle simmer: The water should be steaming and small bubbles should come up from the bottom of the pan. Submerging the lip of each bowl in the simmering water, gently add the eggs, one at a time. Cook for 4 minutes for a soft set, 5 minutes for medium, and 8 minutes for a hard set. Using a slotted spoon, transfer the eggs to a clean dish towel to drain for a minute. Layer the salmon on a plate and place the eggs on top before serving. Garnish with cucumber slices if you are feeling extra fancy or entertaining.

QUICK SALMON SALAD (BHD, FBD)

Prepare and freeze into 6 portions. When you are ready to eat, microwave for less than a minute or let it thaw on the counter for about an hour.

Serves 6

2 lb fresh salmon fillet

2 cups water

1 medium onion

½ cup celery

½ cup fresh parsley

½ cup fresh dill

Juice of 1 lemon

Finely chop onion, celery, parsley, and dill, then mix together in a large bowl. Set aside. Lightly wash the fish. Fill a large, deep skillet with at least 4 inches of water. Add 1 tsp of vinegar per cup of water in the saucepan. Bring to a boil. Reduce to a gentle simmer: The water should be steaming and small bubbles should come up from the bottom of the pan. Add fish and poach for about 6–10 minutes or until fish flakes easily. Remove from heat and drain. Allow fish to cool for about 10 minutes. Afterward, lightly flake the fish with a fork and toss gently with onion mixture. Squeeze lemon juice on top to taste. Serve as an entrée salad on a bed of fresh baby greens or with brown or wild rice.

FRESH MUSHROOM SALAD (BHD, FBD, HHD)

Serves 2

16 oz fresh white mushrooms

1 cup freshly chopped parsley

1 small onion, minced

¼ cup extra virgin olive oil

Juice of 1 lemon

2 cups mixed greens

Wash mushrooms, trim stems, and slice. Place in a large mixing bowl. Coarsely chop fresh parsley and mix with mushrooms. Add minced onion. Whisk the olive oil and lemon juice together and drizzle over mushrooms, then stir to cover completely. Add fresh-ground pepper to taste. Place on top of mixed greens and serve.

OPEN-FACED VEGGIE SANDWICH (BHD, FBD, HHD)

Serves 1

2 slices Ezekiel bread, toasted

½ cucumber, sliced lengthwise

½ fresh tomato, sliced

½ cup spinach leaves

¼ cup canned black beans

¼ cup carrot, grated

1 heaping tbs olive oil mayonnaise

Dash of lemon juice

Mash black beans and lemon juice together. Blend in mayonnaise. Spread bean mixture on each slice of toasted Ezekiel bread. Top with cucumber slices, tomato, spinach leaves, and carrots.

MAZATLAN SHRIMP WITH SALSA (BHD, FBD, HHD)

Serves 8

2 cups diced fresh tomatoes

1 cup chopped red bell pepper

1 cup chopped fresh cilantro

¼ cup diced onion

3 lb fresh shrimp

1 tbs olive oil

Sea salt and pepper to taste

In a large bowl, mix together the diced tomatoes, diced peppers, diced onion, and chopped cilantro. Season lightly with sea salt and black pepper. Let stand in refrigerator. Peel and devein the shrimp. Put olive oil in a large skillet and heat slightly over medium heat. Add shrimp all at once and cook until shrimp are just pink. Spoon salsa mixture over shrimp and serve.

TOMATOES STUFFED WITH CHICKEN SALAD (BHD, FBD, HHD)

Serves 2

¼ cup extra virgin olive oil

1 tbs deli-style mustard

Juice of 1 lemon

2 large tomatoes, ripe, firm

1 tbs minced onion

¼ cup diced celery

¼ cup chopped almonds

3 tbs chopped fresh parsley

8 oz grilled chicken breast, chopped (substitute equal amount of diced tofu for HHD)

Fresh-ground pepper to taste

Combine olive oil, mustard, and lemon juice together to make a dressing and set aside. Cut the tops from the tomatoes and spoon out the flesh and seeds and discard. In a separate mixing bowl, combine chicken, onion, celery, almonds, and 2 tbs of the parsley. Add the dressing and mix well. Fill each hollowed tomato with the mixture and place on platter. Garnish the tops with the remaining 1 tbs of chopped parsley and ground pepper, and serve.

BLACK PEPPER SALMON WITH ASPARAGUS SPEARS (BHD, FBD, HHD)

Serves 6

2½ lb fresh salmon fillets

24 fresh asparagus spears

2 red bell peppers, diced

1 medium yellow onion, diced

Marinade:

¼ cup extra virgin olive oil

¼ cup freshly ground black peppercorns

3 cloves garlic

Juice of ½ lemon

Mix olive oil, garlic, pepper, and lemon juice to form a marinade. Place the salmon in a 1-gallon Ziploc bag and pour marinade over fish. Close tightly and marinate in refrigerator for 1 hour. Meanwhile, mix peppers and onions in bowl and set aside. Preheat oven to 425°F. Wash asparagus spears and place in steamer basket above boiling water. Cover and steam until just tender (6–8 minutes). Place marinated salmon on baking sheet or aluminum foil along with peppers and onions. Bake for 20 minutes or until salmon easily flakes with fork and peppers are just tender. Remove from oven. Divide peppers/ onions into 6 portions and serve with fish and asparagus spears.

NOT SO NAKED CHICKEN (BHD, FBD)

Serves 6

6 5 oz boneless, skinless chicken breasts

1 lemon

2 cloves garlic

½ tsp rosemary

½ tsp thyme

½ tsp oregano

¼ tsp red pepper flakes

¼ tsp paprika

1 tsp extra virgin olive oil

Preheat oven to 350°F. Thoroughly rinse the chicken and pat dry with a paper towel, then place in a baking dish or roasting pan with a lid. Rub the garlic gingerly over the chicken. Rub the olive oil all over the chicken and place it in a roasting pan. Cut a lemon in half and squeeze the juice over the chicken. Mix together the rosemary, thyme, oregano, red chili pepper, and paprika. Sprinkle the mixture over the chicken and cover the pan with lid or aluminum foil. Roast for approximately 45 minutes. Serve with baked sweet potatoes.

QUINOA TABBOULEH (BHD, FBD, HHD)

Serves 4

1 cup quinoa

2 cups water

Salt to taste

1 medium-size ripe tomato, seeded and chopped

¼ cup minced red onion

½ cup canned black beans, rinsed and drained

½ cup fresh parsley, minced

3 tbs chopped mint leaves

⅓ cup extra virgin olive oil

2 tbs fresh lemon juice

Freshly ground black pepper to taste

Wash the quinoa thoroughly to remove any trace of the bitter white coating, then rinse and drain. Bring the water to a boil in a medium-size saucepan. Add salt and quinoa. Reduce the heat to low, cover, and simmer until all the water is absorbed, about 15 minutes. Place the grains in a large serving bowl and set aside to cool. Add the tomatoes, onion, beans, parsley, and mint. In a separate bowl, whisk together the olive oil, lemon juice, and salt and pepper until blended. Pour the dressing over the salad and toss well to combine. Cover and refrigerate for at least 1 hour before serving. Serve chilled.

TURKEY STIR-FRY (BHD, FBD)

Serves 4

2 tsp olive oil

1 lb turkey tenderloin, cut into thin strips

1 cup fat-free chicken broth

4 garlic cloves, minced

¼ tsp crushed red pepper flakes

¼ tsp salt

1 red bell pepper, cut into thin strips

1 cup fresh broccoli florets

1 cup fresh cauliflower florets

2 tbs soy sauce

Place a large nonstick skillet over medium-high heat until hot. Add 1 tsp oil to pan and tilt to coat evenly. Add turkey and stir-fry 5 minutes or until turkey is no longer pink in center. Remove turkey and set aside. Combine broth and garlic, red pepper flakes, and salt. Set aside.

Add remaining 1 tsp oil to pan; add pepper strips, broccoli, and cauliflower; stir-fry 1 minute. Increase heat to high. Stir broth mixture and add to pan with soy sauce, turkey, and any accumulated juices. Bring to a boil; cook 1 to 2 minutes or until slightly thickened. Serve with brown rice.

TEMPEH TAGINE (BHD, FBD, HHD)

Serves 4

1 tsp cumin seeds

1 tsp caraway seeds

1 tsp coriander seeds

½ tsp paprika

½ tsp black peppercorns

1 (1-inch) piece cinnamon stick

2 tsp olive oil

2 cups finely chopped onion

¾ cup finely chopped carrot

½ cup finely chopped celery

½ tsp sea salt

2 garlic cloves, peeled

2 cups (½-inch) cubed peeled sweet potato

2 cups chopped green cabbage

1½ cups water

1 cup finely chopped tomato

1 tbs fresh lemon juice

⅔ cup water

6 tbs fresh lemon juice

⅓ cup finely chopped parsley

2 tsp ground cumin

2 tsp paprika

½ tsp sea salt

½ tsp ground red pepper

4 garlic cloves, minced

1 lb tempeh, cut into ½-inch cubes

To prepare the tagine, combine the first 6 ingredients in a spice or coffee grinder; process until finely ground (you can also use a mortar and pestle if you feel like mashing). Heat oil in a large sauté pan over medium heat. Add onion, carrot, celery, ½ tsp salt, and 2 peeled garlic cloves; cook 5 minutes, stirring occasionally. Cover, reduce heat to low, and cook 20 minutes. Stir in spice mixture, sweet potato, cabbage, water, and tomato; bring to a boil. Reduce heat; simmer, uncovered, 30 minutes or until thick. Stir in lemon juice, and set aside. Then, preheat oven to 350°. Combine ⅔ cup water with all remaining ingredients in a large bowl and toss well to coat. Arrange the tempeh mixture in a single layer in an 11-by-7-inch baking dish. Cover with foil. Bake at 350° for 35 minutes. Uncover and bake an additional 5 minutes or until liquid is absorbed. Serve tempeh over tagine vegetables.

GET CREATIVE!

When I tire of these recipes, and the ones I included in *The Life Plan*, I think about the foods I used to eat and enjoy and try to get creative about cooking them differently so that they are healthier. I'll have Annie find an old recipe that she used to make and replace the unhealthy ingredients with healthy ones. An example would be to substitute pork sausage with veggie sausage, or swap out the cream in one recipe for a vegetable broth. Lots of times, if we can keep the spices the same, the food tastes just as delicious as the more fattening version.

I'll be honest, though, there are some dishes that just don't have a healthy substitution, like one of my all-time favorites, baked macaroni and cheese. Some things we just have to learn to get over and live without. When I really crave it (which is seldom) all I have to do is imagine a big, fat, CLOG in my left main coronary artery, or take a quick look at my "before photos." In about five seconds, the craving is gone.

My Protein Shakes

I'm a big fan of protein shakes. I usually drink them twice a day and count them as meals: one after my morning workout, then a plain chocolate casein protein shake (no fruit) about 30 minutes before bed. They help my body recover from aggressive exercise, restoring muscle glycogen. They also can contribute to muscle repair.

The only time I promote eating a high-glycemic carb is within an hour after aggressive resistance training. Then I'll throw a half banana into an 8- to 10-ounce chocolate protein shake to bump up blood sugars and insulin levels, which will drive amino acids into the muscle tissue. That helps increase muscle tissue and overall strength.

There are tons of different protein shakes on the market, including ones that I sell on my website, www.drlife.com. Although they are all referred to as "protein," they use a wide variety of protein sources, such as whey, casein, egg, soy, and milk. These sources may affect your body differently depending on how fast they are digested. I've found both whey and casein to be smart choices. I like the whey shakes after a workout because they are quickly digested and rapidly provide nutrients to your muscles to promote growth. At night, casein is a better choice because it gets absorbed slowly, so it prevents nighttime munchies.

My shakes make excellent snacks on any of the Life Plan meal plans because they are easy to make and keep you satiated for at least three hours, or until your next meal. They are perfectly apportioned calorie-wise, especially after a long workout. When you are training really hard, you might still be hungry, especially shortly after you work out. The hunger you experience reflects the state of glycogen depletion you have created. This is exactly what you want. As you deplete your muscle and liver glycogen stores, your body is forced to use body fat for its energy, and this is what you need to lose body fat. I view this hunger as a good thing. It tells me that I am burning fat and getting closer to my fat-loss goal. Once I began to think of hunger in a positive way, rather than as something I wanted to avoid, it made it a lot easier to deal with.

However, you don't want to remain hungry for too long, because your body may begin breaking down muscle tissue instead of fat for energy. So, between one to three hours after an intense workout, you should have a protein/carb shake: 0.23 gram of protein and 0.7 gram of a high-glycemic-index carb per pound of body weight. In other words, if you're a 180-pound man, you should consume about 126 grams of carbs and 41 grams of protein. This will quickly replenish your glycogen stores, promote an anabolic hormonal environment for muscle building, and alleviate your hunger. And I would count this as one of your five meals for the day.

The best food to consume immediately after a strength-training workout is 12 ounces of a liquid protein/carbohydrate drink like my shake. And they are very easy to make quickly. You can also make a version of my shake at home using the following ingredients, and blend in a blender for 30–60 seconds to your desired thickness (you may need more ice). When you purchase the whey or casein protein, make sure the ingredients do not include saturated or trans fats:

- 1–2 scoops of a high-quality whey or casein protein

- ½ cup soy milk

- 4 ice cubes

BENEFITS OF WHEY PROTEIN SHAKES

- Absorb quickly

- Digest quickly

- Excellent supplement after aggressive training

BENEFITS OF CASEIN PROTEIN SHAKES

- Absorb slowly

- Digest slowly

- Excellent supplement before bed. Help you sleep because they're slow to digest.

Shake Variations

These small modifications add few calories and lots of flavor. Try them all and then stick with the ones you like best. Remember that the banana versions should be eaten only after a very strenuous workout. Otherwise, follow the directions and skip the banana for a lower glycemic load.

CHOCOLATE PEANUT BUTTER SHAKE

Chocolate protein shake powder (prepare as directed)

1 tbs all-natural peanut butter

Blend in blender with ice.

BERRY BANANA SHAKE

Protein shake powder (plain) (prepare as directed)

1 cup mixed berries (fresh or frozen—no sugar added)

1 small banana

Blend in blender with ice.

BLUEBERRY VANILLA SHAKE

Vanilla protein shake powder (prepare as directed)

½ cup fresh or frozen blueberries (no sugar added)

Blend in blender with ice.

STRAWBERRY BANANA PROTEIN SHAKE

Protein shake powder (plain or vanilla) (prepare as directed)

8–10 fresh strawberries

1 small banana

Blend in blender with ice.

CHOCOLATE ALMOND PROTEIN SHAKE

Chocolate protein shake powder (prepare as directed)

Blend in 1 tbs all-natural almond butter (fresh-ground almonds)

Blend in blender with ice.

CHOCOLATE ALMOND PEANUT BUTTER SHAKE

Chocolate protein shake (prepare as directed)

1 tbs all-natural peanut butter

1 tsp all-natural almond butter

Blend in blender with ice.

When I'm bored with drinking protein shakes, I sometimes add protein powder to my oatmeal in the morning. Heating or cooking the powder unwinds the string of amino acids in the protein molecule and breaks it into smaller pieces. In other words, it starts the digestive process and makes it easier for you to process the amino acids and get them into your bloodstream faster.

Protein shake powder (prepare as directed)   **Blend in blender with ice.**

2 or 3 large eggs whites (boiled)

½ cup steel cut oats, cooked

½ cup berries

FEEDBACK FROM MY FANS

NAME: Ian B.

MESSAGE: Dear Dr. Life, I saw you showing off your book last summer, and being 45 years old thought: If he can do it, so can I! I have lost around 90 pounds following as much of the information I could glean from your book.

My coworkers have seen my success, and the change in energy I have exhibited, and have made me their health guru. I mostly steer them to your book, and give them encouragement. Thank you for sharing the wisdom!

Make Better Choices When Eating Out

It's easier than ever to follow the Life Plan outside your home. The trend today is healthy eating, and it has finally caught on across the country, so much so that even the very best, most exclusive and expensive restaurants can cater to your specific eating requirements. The vast majority of fast-food restaurants also offer a variety of healthier choices on the menu, such as salads and grilled meats.

When Annie and I first met, we used to go out for lunch or dinner all the time, each ordering our own appetizers, main course, and dessert. When I started my transformation, we switched our habits: We'd share an appetizer, then each order an entrée, and then share dessert. That worked, but I realized the portions served at restaurants are simply too large for any one person to finish. Now we each order an appetizer and share one entrée. We find that this provides plenty of food to satisfy our hunger, and at the same time we don't leave the table feeling overfull. On the rare occasions that we do eat dessert, we'll share one, with the goal of leaving half of it on the plate.

The next time you're dining out, remember the following and you'll be able to stick very close to the Life Plan:

- ALWAYS say "NO" to the bread basket.

- ALWAYS ask for water, and drink at least a whole glass before you eat anything. This will help curb your appetite and aid in digesting whatever follows.

- ALWAYS order a fish entrée, and ask for the sauce to be served on the side or not at all—even if you don't see it prepared that way on the menu. If the waitperson says (and I've had this happen), "We can't do substitutions," then very matter-of-factly explain that this is not a substitution at all, just a healthier choice, and you don't want the sauce or butter added. If it's still an issue, just ask to speak with the manager. It's amazing how much attention that grabs.

- ALWAYS order salad dressings served "on the side" and use sparingly.

- Pay careful attention to salad entrées: They often contain far too many calories if they are covered with cheese, bacon, fried chicken, or fish, and of course those creamy dressings.

- Pay careful attention to vegetarian entrées: They can be just as fattening as animal proteins. Avoid high-calorie options that are smothered in cheese or creamy sauces.

- NEVER order any type of sandwich-style entrée. Many times I order a sandwich "without the bread" if there is nothing else on the menu that I can eat.

- NEVER order cream-based soups, breaded or fried foods, or carbonated beverages sweetened with sugar or sugar substitute.

- NEVER order pasta-based entrées: The carb-to-protein ratio will never match what I recommend.

- ALWAYS ask to substitute a side salad with a vinaigrette dressing, or steamed vegetables in place of French fries, potatoes, or rice.

- If the portion looks larger than what you've been eating at home following this program, ask the waiter to bring you a "to go" box and take half off your plate before you start eating.

- NEVER choose buffets or fast-food restaurants where there are too many options and most of them are bad—the more food choices you have the more likely it is that you will eat too much of the wrong foods.

- NEVER order finger foods—nachos, fried cheese sticks, potato skins, even peel-and-eat shrimp. If you can't use a knife and fork, you can't eat with intention and you are more likely to overindulge.

- THE RULE OF TWO: Save your alcoholic consumption for an occasional night out, and limit yourself to TWO of whichever one you want: two glasses of wine, two beers, or two cocktails.

- SKIP dessert, unless they are serving fresh berries.

DEALING WITH CRAVINGS

Think about cravings as your brain's way of telling you it's time to eat. It is not a command to overindulge. When a craving begins, determine how you want to deal with it. It is truly up to you. Remember, a craving is similar to a wave in the ocean. It grows in intensity, peaks, and then subsides if you do not give in. Picture yourself as a surfer who is trying to "ride the wave," instead of being wiped out by it. The more you practice riding the wave, the easier it will become.

Defuse your cravings when you feel them coming on by remembering my "Five Ds":

- DELAY eating anything for at least 10 minutes so that your action is conscious, not impulsive.

- DISTRACT yourself by engaging in an activity that requires concentration, including exercise.

- DISTANCE yourself from food: Get up and go where food is not available.

- DETERMINE how important it really is for you to eat the craved food by taking a quick look at your "before" photo.

- And if all of this fails, then DECIDE what small amount is reasonable and appropriate and eat it very slowly and enjoy! When you are done, ask yourself if it was worth it.

Making It Work

Here are some key rules I try to follow daily that really help me stay on track. They can play an essential role in helping you achieve your goals of leanness, energy, muscularity, and great health.

1. Never forget that everything you put in your mouth can hurt you or help you. This includes alcohol and all wheat products.

2. Make a list of the reasons you want to lose body fat and keep it off forever. Laminate it, carry it in your wallet, and refer to it frequently.

3. Take a "before" picture of yourself with your cell phone and look at it once a day. You'll be surprised just how quickly your body will begin to change.

4. Photocopy the shopping list in Chapter 2 and keep a copy in your wallet. Any one item on that list can be eaten as a snack if you find yourself hungry. In a pinch, go for vegetables first, then fruits, then a protein option.

5. Don't eat unless you are sitting at a table. Your car doesn't count as a table.

6. Avoid eating fast. Savor every bite. Try to spend 15 to 20 minutes eating each and every meal.

7. Avoid fruit juices: They are high in sugar and calories.

8. Choose low-fat or soy options for cheese products if you must have dairy.

9. Don't eat or drink anything for at least two hours before you go to bed except water or a casein shake.

10. Make getting a good night's sleep as much a priority as your eating plan and exercise routine. It is a crucial part of your ability to lose weight and transform your body.

The Life Plan Is Forever

I know all too well that once I reach my fat-loss/muscle-building goals I feel like celebrating. In the past, I'd treat myself to something to eat—something I'd been avoiding. Pretty soon, I found myself returning to my old habits.

If you are anything like me, you will periodically get off track. Make sure that you recognize this right away, and get your act together and get back on the program as soon as possible. Don't wait for "the end of the week" or the start of business on Monday: You don't have this luxury. The more time you spend off track, the harder it will be to get back on. It's truly amazing how little time it takes before we can look just like our "before" photos. That's why this is a forever program. There is no such thing as a separate maintenance program on the Life Plan: Once you reach your goals, keep going. There's always another plateau of better health you can reach, and very likely, it's not far off.

Once you have reached your goals, continue to monitor your body fat percentage, abdominal girth, muscle mass, strength, and all of your biomarkers for disease at least every three months. Get new bathing suit photos of yourself every three months and post them right next to your "before" photo on your refrigerator door, or in your wallet. You don't want to ever forget how you used to look and feel. If you follow these suggestions, I think you will stay on the right track to mastering a lifetime of leanness, great appearance, and great health.

In the next chapter, you'll learn why supplements can be an important part of your personalized program. Remember, they are not a replacement for clean eating: They are a tool to help you get the most out of your diet so that the foods you eat continue to work for you, not against your goals.

CHAPTER 4

Supplementing the Life Plan Diets

- -

A s anyone who's spent more than 10 minutes on the Internet knows, supplements are a booming business. They are advertised everywhere, and even some of the most reputable doctors are pitching them. But are supplements safe and do they have proven efficacy—or are they just marketing hype?

The answer is a firm "maybe," which is nothing if not frustrating. The variability among producers, brand names, and even types of supplements can make even the most levelheaded man's brain burst. So let me give you a quick run-through of all of your different options, and then I'll focus on the few that I find to be the most effective.

Types of Supplementation
- -

There are two major groups of supplements. The first I'll refer to as *essential nutrients*, which are replacements for crucial vitamins and minerals that your body must have in order to function properly. These include vitamins and minerals, essential fatty acids, and probiotics.

Vitamins are organic compounds, meaning that they come from living things, like plants or animals. They are necessary for proper bodily functioning, and we need only very small amounts of them. However, our bodies cannot manufacture sufficient quantities of them on our own. Instead, we have to get them from the foods we eat. In order to ensure that people get the right amounts of certain vitamins, the U.S. government requires that some processed foods be fortified with vitamins. These include milk and dairy products, breakfast cereals, and grains.

Minerals are inorganic elements that come from the soil and water and are then absorbed by plants or animals that we eat. Our bodies need large amounts of some minerals, such as calcium, and very small amounts of other minerals, such as selenium and chromium, to stay healthy.

Essential fatty acids (EFAs) are compounds that are necessary for optimal health, yet we cannot make them in our bodies and must, therefore, consume them from high-fat foods. There are two basic types: omega-6 fatty acids found in cooking oils, and omega-3 fatty acids found in fatty fish and some plants. Omega-3 fatty acids have anti-inflammatory effects and are helpful for combating inflammatory diseases such as rheumatoid arthritis. They are also considered protective against heart disease. Americans consume roughly 10 times more omega-6 fatty acids than omega-3 fatty acids. These large amounts of omega-6 fatty acids produce an unhealthy imbalance in the omega-3 to omega-6 fatty acid ratio, which is thought to be a contributing factor for heart and blood vessel disease. To strike a better balance, we need to increase our consumption of omega-3 fatty acids, and one way to do this is through dietary supplements of high-quality fish oil capsules.

Probiotics are living microorganisms similar to what is normally found in the human gut. They are also referred to as "friendly bacteria" or "good bacteria." Probiotics may help with a number of health issues, including GI distress, symptoms of lactose intolerance, inflammation, cancer prevention, and enhanced micronutrient absorption.

Of these four categories, only some vitamins and probiotics are found in the body, although as we get older, we tend to produce smaller quantities. Yet all four types of essential nutrients are necessary to good health. Supplementing these nutrients has been studied in both short-term and longitudinal research and has demonstrated overwhelming efficacy for a variety of health concerns. For example, a vitamin D deficiency is linked to all kinds of accelerated aging; fish oil supplementation reduces your risk for vascular disease leading to heart attacks and strokes; and many vitamins work together to improve immune function and protect the body against many cancers.

Several years ago scientists thought that supplementing with vitamins and minerals was necessary only to prevent such diseases as scurvy, pellagra, and rickets—diseases we rarely hear about today. Now nutritional experts fully understand that these same micronutrients play key roles in the prevention of heart disease, cancer, arthritis, and cataracts, along with the signs and symptoms of aging, including loss of muscle mass, strength, and bone mass. Supplementing your diet guarantees that you have every advantage in order to optimize health, fight disease, improve libido, sharpen the mind, stabilize blood sugar/insulin, and maintain energy levels so that you can work out vigorously and still have plenty of stamina for the rest of the day.

Regardless of how healthily we eat, supplementing with quality nutraceuticals is critical for everybody, especially men. Soils have long been depleted of vitamins and minerals from years of overfarming, chemical toxins, and acid rain. And, even if they eat only organic foods that are thought to be higher in vitamins and minerals, most men do not consume sufficient amounts of the many nutrients we need from the foods we eat, even if we follow a careful diet, such as the Life Plan. On top of that, men who push their bodies hard with aerobic and resistance training exercises definitely need additional nutritional support. During exercise, your sweat is detoxing your system, and as you lose water, you are also losing essential nutrients. We also require increased amounts of vitamins and minerals to make sure our metabolic machinery runs at peak performance to support our workouts.

Oxidative stress is another very important reason active men need to make sure that they are getting the right amount of micronutrients. Oxidation is the term used for the process of removing electrons from an atom or molecule. The result of this change can be destructive: For example, rust occurs on iron as it is exposed to oxygen. The same process can occur throughout the body. As we create energy by burning digested food with the oxygen we breathe, this process enables us to create a lean, muscular, healthy body. However, excess oxygen can produce dangerous by-products, which include free radicals. Free radicals are the electronically unstable oxygen molecules that must scavenge electrons from whatever sources they can to become stable molecules. The sources of these scavenged electrons can include DNA, cell membranes, important enzymes, and vital structural or functional proteins. When these important cell parts and substances lose their electrons to these free radicals, their function is altered, and the results can be catastrophic—cancer, heart disease, dementia, arthritis, muscle damage, increased susceptibility to infection, and accelerated aging. And while the Life Plan workouts are making you healthier, the program is working against you in terms of free-radical formation: Working out for at least five hours per week can greatly increase the risk of your body tissues suffering from excess free radicals.

The good news is that the fix is relatively easy. Antioxidants found in colorful fruits and vegetables can help protect us from these free radicals. Supplementation with relatively high doses of the known antioxidants, which include vitamins C, E, and A, the mineral selenium, and phytochemicals, is probably the most reasonable way to address this issue. Antioxidants will not only help prevent the degenerative diseases I described above, they will also speed up your recovery from high-intensity workouts, promote muscle and strength building, and prevent exercise-related muscle injuries.

However, when it comes to taking supplemental vitamins, more is not always better. Some vitamins are actually dangerous if consumed in high dosages. For example, too much vitamin A can lead to toxicity and bone loss. Some are more effective when they are kept refrigerated, including probiotics such as acidophilus. And some may interact with medications that you are currently taking, such as blood thinners. Always work with your doctor to determine the right levels for you. Start the discussion by mentioning the range I suggest below and tailor it to your current weight and health status. Make sure your doctor knows all of your medications and that you are planning on following an intense exercise and nutrition program.

Remember, vitamins and minerals cannot cure a disease, so they are not a substitute for prescription medications that you may be taking. Rather, they bolster your body's overall function so that, over time, you may be able to lower the dosage of or eliminate some of your prescription drugs. For example, folate, better known as folic acid, is one of the B vitamins and is necessary for the healthy division of cells and the prevention of colon cancer. It can play a key role in the growth of new muscle tissue that is essential to increasing muscle mass and strength. It also helps prevent heart and blood vessel disease by keeping homocystine levels low. A large government study in 2002 found that people who consumed the most folate had the fewest strokes and least amount of heart disease. This doesn't mean, however, that these people were able to stop taking their medication.

How to Choose the Right Vitamins
- -
Contrary to what most men believe, the supplement industry actually does have to follow some federal regulations, but not to the degree that the pharmaceutical industry does. At the same time, the FDA acknowledges that it has limited resources, in relation to the supplement industry's size, for adequately enforcing regulations. They are supposed to regulate the manufacturing processes and market claims, focusing on labeling and product marketing (performed in conjunction with the FTC). For example, use of the term "Dietary Supplement" and claims of health benefits are regulated and defined by the FDA. Yet the terms "nutraceuti-

cal" and "functional food" are not regulated. New dietary ingredients don't have to be tested or registered before marketing. Perhaps most important, a supplement will be removed from the market shelves only after a product has proven to be unsafe.

When you are purchasing supplements, I recommend that you always look for high-quality, pharmaceutical-grade products. The supplement must be 99 percent pure and free of fillers, binders, and unknown substances, and pass a rigorous approval procedure by the United States Pharmacopeia (USP). Look for the words "USP approved" on labels or product information websites or pamphlets: This provides assurance to the consumer that the quality and purity of raw materials used in the manufacture of each supplement are of pharmaceutical grade and guarantees a certain standard of excellence.

There are several excellent-quality vitamin and mineral supplement lines available. Cenegenics nutraceuticals are high-quality, pharmaceutical-grade products that I recommend. Dr. Kenneth H. Cooper has also created a line of excellent vitamin and mineral supplements. These products can be reviewed on his website, www.coopercomplete.com.

One of his products is called Cooper Complete Elite Athlete formulation. This is a vitamin/mineral supplement designed specifically for the high-endurance aerobic athletes, but I believe that it works equally well for anyone involved in high-intensity resistance training. It does lack calcium, so be sure you add a 1,000- or 1,200-milligram supplement to your regimen if you take this product. Less expensive products that have decent quality include Vita Smart Multi-Vitamins Men's and One A Day 50 Plus.

Nutraceuticals

The second type of supplement group is now commonly referred to as *nutraceuticals*. This term was coined to refer to foods, or parts of food, including dietary supplements, that provide medical or health benefits, including the prevention and treatment of disease, in addition to its basic nutritional value. This category covers a wide swath, from energy bars and drinks to nutritional supplements in the forms of botanicals, teas, spices, and herbs, as well as compounds and formulations of dietary supplements. Though there have been many studies that can support the effectiveness of nutraceuticals, there have been an equal number that show these to be less than effective. Because of this, I'm cautious about many of these types of supplements. I feel comfortable recommending the ones I've listed below, as they have been shown to have some proven efficacy.

As with essential nutrients, the quality of nutraceuticals varies greatly. Many are produced overseas where there is a complete lack of regulation. Therefore, I suggest that you look for products made in the United States whenever possible. And while their names sound quite benign, they actually can cause dangerous and adverse reactions when combined with prescription medication. Therefore, I also suggest that you talk with your doctor before taking any type of nutraceutical.

The Life Plan Supplement Shopping List

Here are my suggestions for supplements that every active man needs in order to optimize his health and quality of life. You can adapt this list based on your current health and your own doctor's recommendations.

It's best to split your daily supplements into a morning dose and an evening dose because this allows your body to maintain a sufficient level of the water-soluble antioxidants needed to fight off free radicals. It really doesn't matter which ones you take in the morning or evening. Most comprehensive multivitamins/minerals are packaged in such a way that you take one serving in the morning and the other in the evening. I divide my fish oil into a morning serving and an evening serving. Melatonin should be taken at night because it enhances sleep. Some of my patients think vitamin D3 also helps them achieve a more restful sleep. As you read through the details for each of these supplement suggestions, you'll also see how they work together, and which should be taken at the same time.

1. Essential nutrient: comprehensive multivitamin and mineral supplement
2. Essential nutrient: essential fatty acids
3. Essential nutrient: probiotic supplement
4. Essential nutrient: vitamin D3
5. Essential nutrient: calcium
6. Nutraceutical: CoQ_{10}
7. Nutraceutical: saw palmetto
8. Nutraceutical: lycopene
9. Nutraceutical: milk thistle
10. Nutraceutical: pycnogenol/L-arginine

Comprehensive Multivitamin and Mineral Supplement

Every man needs a good multivitamin and mineral supplement every day: Consider these to be the most essential nutrients. Multivitamin capsules are digested and metabolized faster than tablets. Make sure you pick one that has at least 100 percent of the Recommended Dietary Allowances (RDA) for thiamin (B1), riboflavin (B2), niacin (B3), vitamins B6, B12, E, linoleic acid, and folic acid. You also need 2,000 milligrams of vitamin C, at least 400 IU of vitamin E, and at least 100 mg of magnesium. Your multivitamin should also contain at least 20 mcg of vitamin K, as well as the minerals chromium, copper, selenium, and zinc (15 mg). If you are on a blood thinner (such as Coumadin), talk with your doctor about how much vitamin K you require.

Vitamin A toxicity can easily be avoided by simply taking beta-carotene, which your body converts to vitamin A. Beta-carotene doesn't cause bone loss, but too much beta-carotene may increase the risk of lung cancer if you are a smoker (which you shouldn't be, but you know that already). You don't need more than 15,000 IU daily of beta-carotene. The vitamin A in supplements can also come from retinol (often called vitamin A palmitate or acetate). To protect your bones, limit retinol to no more than 3,000 IU per day.

Essential Fatty Acids

My minimum recommendation for this essential nutrient is 300–500 mg daily. Purchase high-quality fish oil supplements that have the highest amount of eicosapentaenoic acid, EPA, and docosahexanoic acid, DHA, per capsule, and keep them refrigerated. You need to take four one-gram capsules daily in order to create the best balance for your body. The content of high-quality fish oil should be made up of at least 60 percent of both essential fatty acids (EPA and DHA) combined. The concentration of DHA should not be less than 18 percent, and a higher concentration is a signal of superior quality. EFAs show strong evidence for use as anti-inflammatories and in the promotion of overall health.

The highest-quality fish oil supplements are made in New Zealand and Norway. Oily fish found in these regions of the world are less contaminated by pollutants than similar fish found in other regions of the world. Consequently, the oil obtained from them does not require as much purification. Always read the list of ingredients found on the bottle. If additives or preservatives have been added to increase shelf life, they might make the overall supplement less effective. Ultrarefined and ultrapurified fish oil products are better choices because they typically are made from pharmaceutical-grade fish oil. Look for labels that indicate that the product has undergone "molecular distillation," which not only removes mercury and dioxin impurities but also balances out the concentration of other nutrients, such as vitamin A and D, if present.

VITAMIN E GOES WITH FISH OIL

Because fish oil does not compensate for potential oxidative damage, it's also a good idea to increase your intake of vitamin E. I recommend that you take between 400 and 800 IU of vitamin E per day. While some fish oil capsules, as well as your multivitamin, may also contain some vitamin E, it may not be enough.

If you take cod liver oil (some men prefer this to fish oil capsules), be aware that it also contains vitamins A and D. Depending on how much cod liver oil you use and what other supplements you're taking, you could be getting too much of these vitamins. An alternative is devitaminized cod liver oil.

Probiotic Supplement

Probiotic supplements are considered essential nutrients and are available as capsules, powders, and tablets. I think it is prudent to include probiotics in your daily regimen because they are thought to enhance fat metabolism, stimulate mineral absorption, improve GI function, and multiply "healthy" bacteria in the intestine. Choose one that is a blend of at least six "live" cultures and that is kept in a refrigerated case, and make sure to keep them refrigerated at home. Follow the manufacturer's recommended dosing on the label since dosage can differ, depending on the probiotic source.

Vitamin D3

Vitamin D is really not a vitamin at all: It's a hormone. Yet it is still considered an essential nutrient in my book. Adequate vitamin D levels can protect you against cancer, infections, and premature aging. Vitamin D helps your body absorb calcium and is vital for skeletal development/ health and prevention of osteoporosis. Vitamin D deficiency/insufficiency is also a risk factor for cardiovascular disease, hypertension, and Type 2 diabetes. A June 2008 study reported that vitamin D deficiency gives men a 2.5 times higher risk for heart attack. They also found that men with intermediate vitamin D levels demonstrated a 60 percent increased myocardial infarction risk. For all of these reasons, I believe that it is critical that every man gets enough D.

Most men who work indoors have insufficient or deficient levels of vitamin D, because it is mostly (90 percent) manufactured in our skin when we are exposed to sunlight. Eating vitamin D–rich foods cannot solve the problem alone. If you live in the northern third of the United States, Canada, or Alaska you're probably not getting enough vitamin D during the winter months. This, combined with the fact that most winter activity is limited to the indoors, results in many men having very little sun exposure.

Vitamin D supplementation is particularly important for overweight African-American men. African-Americans have multiple risk factors for cardiovascular disease. According to Ryan A. Harris, Ph.D., assistant professor at the Georgia Prevention Institute at Georgia Health Sciences University, African-Americans are more likely than people of other races to develop Type 2 diabetes, and when they develop high blood pressure it tends to be more severe as compared to other groups. African-Americans also have a greater risk of developing vitamin D deficiency because their skin pigmentation inhibits the skin cells' ability to produce vitamin D in response to exposure to sunlight.

A blood test for 25-hydroxy-vitamin D is the best way to determine your status. Levels less than 30 ng/mL are considered to be a deficiency state. Optimal levels are 60 to 90 ng/mL. Most of my patients need to take 5,000 IU to 10,000 IU daily to achieve these levels, which is significantly less than what is offered in even the best multivitamin. Choose a supplement containing cholecalciferol (D3), and make sure to talk to your doctor about vitamin D supplementation if you are currently taking antiseizure medications.

Calcium

Calcium is the most abundant mineral in the body. It is naturally found in some foods and added to others, such as milk products. It is also available as a dietary supplement and present in most antacids. Calcium supplementation is essential for bone health.

Calcium is required for muscle contraction, blood vessel expansion and contraction, secretion of hormones and enzymes, and transmitting impulses throughout the nervous system. The body strives to maintain constant concentrations of calcium in blood, muscle, and intercellular fluids. When our intake of calcium is low, the body willfully pulls calcium from bones in order to maintain critical concentrations. Then, as we age, our weakened bones can break down due to calcium loss, resulting in osteoporosis.

Calcium requires its own set of pills, because you need 1,000 to 1,200 mg daily, which is far less than what is available in a typical multivitamin. The two main forms of calcium found in supplements are calcium carbonate and calcium citrate. Calcium carbonate is more commonly available and is both inexpensive and convenient. Both the carbonate and citrate forms are similarly well absorbed, but men taking medications such as Pepcid that reduce levels of stomach acid can absorb calcium citrate more easily.

Coenzyme Q_{10}

Coenzyme Q_{10} is a nutraceutical that I can stand behind. It is actually a vitaminlike chemical that is found in practically all the cells in the body, especially the heart. It has antioxidant properties, and the body uses it to generate ATP, the cellular storage unit of energy. Coenzyme Q_{10} levels start declining after the age of 20. Low levels of CoQ_{10} are thought to interfere with energy production pathways in our body.

The potential benefits of taking CoQ_{10} include antioxidant activity, prevention of age-related macular degeneration, enhancing athletic performance, improved immune function, prevention of heart disease, and slowing the aging process. Any man who is taking a statin drug to control cholesterol levels must take extra Coenzyme Q_{10} because statins deplete CoQ_{10} from skeletal and cardiac muscle. The recommended dose of Coenzyme Q_{10} is 100 mg if you are not on a statin and 200 mg daily if you are on a statin. Choose the form of CoQ_{10} called ubiquinol, which is the electron-rich form of this supplement and is used more efficiently by our bodies.

Saw Palmetto

Saw palmetto is another proven nutraceutical that is used mainly for relieving urinary symptoms associated with an enlarged prostate gland (benign prostatic hyperplasia, or BPH), such as frequent nighttime urination. Several small studies suggest that saw palmetto may be effective for treating BPH symptoms. However, a 2009 review of the research concluded that saw palmetto has not been shown to be more effective than a placebo for this use.

My experience is mixed; I believe it has significantly helped reduce the number of times I have to get up at night. Others feel it hasn't helped them much. I think it's worthwhile to give it a try, since it is well tolerated by most men. Look for a supplement that is standardized to contain 85 to 95 percent fatty acids and sterols. Recommended dose is 160 mg twice a day.

Lycopene

Lycopene is a phytochemical nutraceutical that creates the bright red pigment found in tomatoes and other red fruits and vegetables, such as watermelons and papayas (but not strawberries or cherries). Research indicates men who get more lycopene in their diet have a reduced risk of prostate cancer. Other research suggests lycopene supplementation inhibits progression of benign prostatic hyperplasia. It also has beneficial antioxidant effects.

I think it is prudent to take 20 mg daily of this nutrient. Compare this dosage to the ingredients in your multivitamin to ensure that you are covered: Many multis include lycopene as well. It is better absorbed when taken with a fatty acid, so make sure to take it at the same time as your fish oil supplements.

Milk Thistle

The seeds of the milk thistle have been used for over 2,000 years to treat chronic liver disease and protect the liver against toxins. It may also be useful in the prevention and treatment of prostate cancer. Look for a standardized extract of this nutraceutical that contains 70 percent silymarin at the dose of 200 mg twice a day.

Pycnogenol Plus L-arginine

Great sex requires a strong erection, which relies on the relaxation of the cavernous smooth muscle and dilation of blood vessels, which are triggered by the chemical nitric oxide (NO). Pycnogenol, a natural plant extract from the bark of the maritime pine tree, increases the production of your own nitric oxide. When Pycnogenol is combined with L-arginine, it has been shown to produce a significant improvement in sexual function in men with erectile dysfunction (ED), without any side effects. The best dose is 40 mg of Pycnogenol, two times a

---

ASK DR. LIFE

QUESTION FROM BILL M.: I've heard you talk about how dangerous belly fat is as a risk factor for heart disease. Are there any supplements that can really help me lose my belly?

ANSWER: Bill, the time-proven way to get rid of abdominal fat is to combine a restricted caloric nutritional program with a consistent exercise program using both high-intensity resistance and aerobic training. Some researchers believe that supplementing with branched-chain amino acids such as leucine, isoleucine, and valine is an additional strategy to target troublesome fat, especially around the belly. These nutrients are the major building blocks for muscle tissue that play a critical role in regulating metabolism during exercise. When added to a solid nutritional/exercise program, supplementing with these amino acids can help tap into the intra-abdominal fat stores for energy . . . stores that ordinarily are reserved until all other sources are depleted. They may just give you that extra edge to get rid of your spare tire. But supplements are never enough: You have to do the hard work in the gym, too.

day, and 2 g of L-arginine, once a day. I have personally used this combination of supplements and can attest to its effectiveness for men with or without ED.

The Truth about Fat Burners and Muscle Builders

In general, I'm not a huge fan. Most sports enhancers are typically more hype than hard truth. They certainly don't do the work for you: You still need to get out and get sweaty in order to get the results that you are looking for. However, they are on the market, and if you are going to try one, I suggest that you try something that is as safe as possible.

HMB (hydroxy-methylbutyrate) is a relatively new ingredient that men are talking about in terms of its ability to burn fat and build muscle. It is a by-product of the amino acid leucine and is naturally found in only two types of food: catfish and grapefruit. It is also produced by the human body. HMB is an active ingredient in the popular Ensure product line: It is found in those drinks labeled "Revigor." Three other companies currently market the product as a dietary supplement.

Although it has not been widely studied, researchers claim that HMB enhances the gains in muscle strength and lean mass associated with resistance training by making proteins more available to the body, particularly after a workout. In doing so, HMB allows athletes to retain more protein in their system, resulting in increased energy levels and faster recovery. When we ingest extra amounts of HMB, it acts as a performance enhancer for such activities as weight lifting and sprinting by boosting strength levels, enhances gains in muscle size and strength, and prevents postworkout muscle tissue breakdown. There have been no studies that contradict these findings.

Putting It All Together

You now have everything you need to master the Life Plan in terms of food and nutrition. Stay on script for at least three weeks before you make any changes to your diet, or even move from one level to another. You need to give your body and metabolism a little bit of time to adjust to these changes, especially if they are drastically different from what you've been eating in the past. If you are following this program religiously, you should see a change on the scale within the first two weeks.

You can consult my previous book, *The Life Plan*, for more details on the eating program and different food options. However, you'll find that the shopping list is pretty much the same as what we have here, and maybe even a little more restrictive.

Use the journal in Chapter 8 to start recording your own transformation, and carefully keep track of what you eat every day. That way you'll have a clear record of how you were able to achieve good results. You'll also be able to determine if any type of food affects you negatively, and once you pinpoint that information, you can avoid that food in the future.

The next challenge for you to master is the Life Plan workouts. This is the fun part of the program, and the area that will allow you to make real and lasting changes to the way you look. The truth is, you can diet all you want, but if you don't work out, you can't really redefine your body. I'm not going to lie to you: The following workouts are going to be tough at first. But I can also promise that if you stick with it, you'll like the way you look, maybe for the first time in a long while.

MEET BRADLEY

When I was first evaluated by Dr. Life, I was an achy, tired 51-year-old who had a five-year-old daughter whom I couldn't keep up with. Even though I had been a personal trainer back in the 1980s and exercise was always part of my life, some days I felt like I was 75 years old. This program makes me feel like I am back in my 30s again, and I attribute that to the consistent use of high-quality supplements.

Before I met Dr. Life another doc had me taking baby aspirin every day to prevent heart disease. Dr. Life suggested that I take a multivitamin, DHEA, fish oil, and vitamin D. He explained how all of these were important, and that I couldn't possibly get them from my diet. I didn't think much of it, but I realized that I'm taking these nutrients that my body needs to perform and heal itself, and in combination with revitalizing my exercise program, it began to completely change the way I felt.

Two and a half years later I still feel great, and I think that's because I've been very consistent. I hardly remember how bad I felt before. The proof is in the bloodwork: The areas that we needed to improve have in fact improved, and the scores are right there in the blood test report. My blood chemistry is amazing, and as a personal trainer, I know that by nourishing my body it's making my workouts more effective. It's all a part of the same process.

PART TWO

MASTERING THE LIFE PLAN WORKOUTS

CHAPTER 5

The Life Plan Flexibility, Core, and Balance Workout

Flexibility is defined by the ease with which you can move all the joints—your fingers, hands, wrists, elbows, knees, hips, feet, toes, neck, and spine—freely through a full range of motion and without pain. The ability to remain flexible is much the same as having good bone density or muscle mass: It's a "use it or lose it" situation. In order to "use it" you need to be able to comfortably twist, bend, turn, and reach. Yet as we age, flexibility can become an issue, and stiffness in the joints or back pain often settles in. Many inactive men experience the same symptoms that I had: tightness in the legs and lower back. This occurs because we spend the majority of our adult lives standing around, or worse, sitting. Unless you're in the habit of moving your legs and lower back, everything will eventually tighten up.

Loss of flexibility can also lead to balance issues. Tight muscles and joints force the body into faulty movement patterns, lousy posture, and overall instability. When your body has to compensate for muscle tightness, it sends distorted signals to your brain from your sensory nervous system, which then triggers your body to recruit other muscles so that you can perform a particular movement. For example, if your chest is tight it will cause your shoulders to round. This change throws off your body's alignment, and you will be off balance.

All of the systems related to balance decline with aging—if we let them. These include touch and pressure sensation on the bottoms of your feet, vision (both acuity and edge detection), proprioception (sensory information that provides feedback to your brain about joint position and movement), and vestibular input (the sense of body movement located in our inner ear). A loss of strength also affects balance. However, when you combine flexibility exercises with balance training, you create an exercise practice that will keep you on your feet and delay feeling old.

FLEXIBILITY AND SEX?

You bet! A flexible man is a sexual man. And if you won't take my word for it, consult the Kama Sutra.

I've also found that improving my flexibility has helped me lower my stress levels. When I was inflexible I could feel the tightness throughout my body, and this, at an unconscious level, made me feel stressed out. The tighter I got the more stressed I felt. As my flexibility has improved I have noticed less tightness and stress, and I sleep better, which makes me feel healthier and gives me the ability to be more active. In short, being able to move around without pain and having a full range of motion promotes a healthier lifestyle: If you feel better, you'll look better, and you'll be better.

The benefits of flexibility and balance training include:

- A more youthful gait

- Improved coordination

- Improved posture

- Improved reaction time

- Improved sexual function

- Increased range of motion

- Reduced lower back pain

- Reduced muscle soreness

- Reduced risk of muscle injury

- Reduced risks of falling

Pilates Is the Perfect Flexibility Practice

When I was writing *The Life Plan* I had just begun exploring Pilates training. Since then, I've fully embraced the technique. It is by far the fastest way I have found to improve flexibility and balance, and I can link this exercise to the dramatic improvement in my posture, gait, and agility. Today I move more rapidly and more youthfully than I did in my thirties. Pilates has helped me make my body more fluid by targeting stiff muscles and joints while enhancing core strength and spinal health. I've learned that when you have a stronger core, you can move more freely. It has also helped protect me from injuries and has increased my overall strength, two important factors that allow me to have a rigorous resistance-training workout every day, which is what ultimately helps me burn the most calories and maintain leanness.

The Pilates technique was developed by trainer/gymnast Joseph Pilates back in 1926. Today, Pilates is one of the fastest-growing exercise methods in the world. The exercises emphasize an awareness of proper breathing and the right spinal/pelvic alignment. The workouts are performed either on a mat using your body as resistance weight, or on specially designed resistance-based equipment.

When I first started a few years ago, I had to follow a very modified practice because I was so inflexible. Over time I've been able to broaden my range of exercises. But the result I'm most proud of in terms of this practice is how it has helped my overall posture. When I first started working with my trainer, Shane Gagne, she told me that I was walking around like an old man. I was always leaning forward with rounded shoulders, and my gaze went to the floor instead of up and out. Today, my posture has changed greatly, and I'm much more aware of what my body is doing and what it is capable of.

I also feel as if I gained a little bit of height, even though it's not exactly true. Men do get physically smaller as they age and the spinal discs compress. Pilates has helped elongate my muscles so that I can stand more erect, and now I have the appearance of being taller. If you measure your height now before you start this practice, you may actually see an increase in height over time, but it's actually taking you back to how tall you were in your thirties, before you began to shrink and stoop.

I recommend that you follow this workout at least three times a week, but you can do Pilates every day, because you're not tearing down muscle, you're toning, strengthening, and lengthening the muscles you already have. Because of this, you don't need the same type of resting period that comes with weight-lifting or resistance training.

A typical workout takes 50 minutes to an hour, and if you are a beginner, it may take even longer. As you get better, the workout actually gets shorter, or you can add new movements to make the routine more challenging. There are over 500 Pilates exercises that can be performed on special machines, like the Pilates Reformer, or on the floor. While you might not have access to this special equipment, I've created the following Pilates routine to be a total floor workout: You can do this right in your own home, at the gym, or when you are traveling. Even though I prefer to use the Reformer, as pictured below, you can do these same exercises right on a clean, level floor.

This routine can be followed by anyone: A beginner would probably find it a little bit difficult at first; intermediates will still find it challenging, and advanced individuals with no physical issues can use this as a starting point or refresher to their practice.

Pilates can be performed during any part of your day. Some people like to do it before other types of exercise; others like to do it at the end of the day to wind down. Because I do it daily as part of my complete exercise routine (along with cardio and resistance training), I like to do it after my resistance training but before cardio. I enjoy this balance because the weight-lifting is building and strengthening muscle; the Pilates helps keep me lean and at the same time is making sure that I don't get stiff after my workout. On the days that you'll be doing all three types of exercise, I recommend this format.

Pilates classes are held in many gyms and private studios throughout the country. For the complete beginner, I recommend that you take a couple of classes so that you can learn the basic technique with a trained instructor watching over you, because you'll have a hard time determining if you are performing the movements correctly. Every class is different and every teacher is different, but the movements remain the same. And one of the nicest aspects of Pilates is that all the exercises can be modified so anybody can do them, regardless of level of expertise. So don't be afraid to walk into a class; everyone in there is working at his or her own level. Then, once you get the postures and techniques down, you can do it on your own.

Tips to Make Your Practice Perfect
- -

- During the workout you'll be holding each stretch for about 30 seconds, and you may feel some level of discomfort. If you're in the middle of a stretch and you're feeling a lot of pain, or more pain than you're comfortable with, stop the movement immediately and assess the problem. There's always a level of discomfort that comes with deep stretching, but you should never feel a sharp pain or a sense of searing, burning, or tingling.

- If you have a fever or are feeling nauseated, dizzy, lightheaded, or short of breath you shouldn't be doing Pilates. Take the day off.

- If you're sore from another activity or injury, use caution. My general belief is that movement is always better than no movement, but don't push yourself to the point of significant pain.

- I recommend a light meal before a Pilates workout. You don't want to eat anything too heavy before exercising, but you wouldn't want to be empty-bellied either, because you can become dizzy and lightheaded. Sometimes I have a piece of fruit, such as an apple, or a small portion of oatmeal before my practice.

- Communicate with your instructor if you have any kind of restrictions, injuries, or illness so he or she can modify the exercise.

- Breathe in through the nose and out through the mouth, and continue to breathe even while you are holding your stretch. Breathe from your diaphragm by allowing your belly to extend, instead of your chest, on every inhalation; your belly should draw in during every exhalation.

- Always eat after the workout. You can have a protein shake or an apple, depending on how you feel. You need to replenish because you do burn more calories in Pilates than you would expect. The typical caloric deficit in a one-hour session is roughly 300-plus calories.

- Even if you're not sweating a lot, drink some water during and certainly after class.

- Wear comfortable clothing that is not too loose. You might want to wear compression shorts underneath regular gym shorts for more support. You will be taking off your shoes, but keep your socks on.

- The room you're using should be kept cool.

- You will need a Thera-Band and a clean towel. A Thera-Band is a latex exercise band that is available at most sports equipment stores, Pilates studios, or on the Internet. They come in eight color-coded levels of resistance.

- The more you stretch the quicker you will see the results. Stretch during commercial breaks while watching television, using any of the stretches below.

Dr. Life's Pilates Routine

The flexibility exercises outlined below allow you to engage in deep stretching, which teaches your body to move without restraint so that you will prevent and reverse muscular pain. You typically hold each stretch for at least 30 seconds in order to get the stretch flex to relax. The stretch flex is the contraction of a muscle in response to a sudden, brisk, longitudinal stretching of the same muscle. During Pilates we do not bounce during the stretching because that risks muscle tearing. The program is fluid: You will go from one exercise right into the next without resting. During the exercises, most people feel pretty comfortable and are not sweating excessively.

Be patient during your stretches and do not force joints to go farther than they want.

Severe pain while stretching is a signal that the stretch has gone too far. Mild to moderate pain during a stretch indicates you are doing the stretch properly to make advances. There should be no soreness the next day after a stretching routine; if there is it is an indication that you have overstretched and should lower the intensity of stretching the next time you perform them. This can be done by not stretching the muscle so far or not holding the stretch as long.

Breathe slowly, and never hold your breath while stretching. Proper breathing helps relax your body, increases blood flow throughout your body, and helps mechanically remove lactic acid and other by-products of exercise.

Exercise 1: HAMSTRING STRETCH

Stretching the hamstrings elongates the leg muscles. The stretch should be felt through the back.

To start: Sit on the floor with a Thera-Band or on a Pilates Reformer as pictured.

Instructions:

1. Put the Thera-Band around your left foot. Grab the ends of the Thera-Band so you can stretch your leg. Lie on your back with the left leg extended up to the ceiling, and

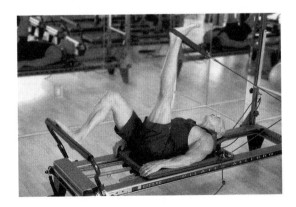

square off your hips. Anchor your lower back to the floor. Don't arch your neck or lift your head off the floor.

2. Using the resistance of the Thera-Band, pull your leg toward the body for a bigger stretch. Reach your heel out of your hips for more control and to increase the stretch.

3. Relax and repeat on your right leg. Repeat for a total of 10 stretches on each leg.

Exercise 2: PIRIFORMIS STRETCH

This stretch works the piriformis, the muscle located on the upper part of the buttocks. It is tight in almost everybody who doesn't actively stretch it on a regular basis.

To start: Lying on the floor, cross your left ankle to the right knee.

Instructions:

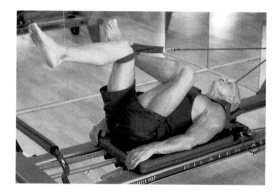

1. With your hands, grasp under your right knee and pull toward your body, stretching the hip.

2. Relax and repeat on the right leg. Repeat for a total of 10 stretches on each leg.

VARIATION: You can also do this stretch sitting in a chair: Cross one ankle to the opposite knee and lean forward over the leg. Repeat for a total of 10 stretches on each leg.

Exercise 3: STANDING QUAD STRETCH

To start: Stand, holding on to a stable surface for balance.

Instructions:

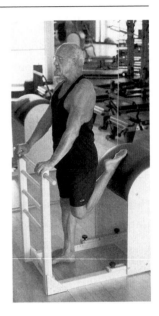

1. Bend your left knee, bringing the heel of your foot to your buttocks, and grasp the front of your foot with your hand.

2. Pull your heel to your buttocks and lengthen the front of your hip to stretch your quad muscle.

3. Relax and repeat on your right leg. Repeat for a total of 10 stretches on each leg.

Exercise 4: QUAD STRETCH

To start: Lie on the right side of your body.

Instructions:

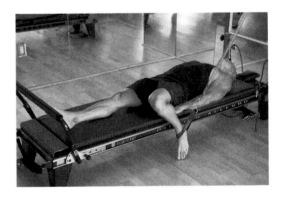

1. Bend your left knee, bringing the heel of your left foot to your buttocks to stretch the quad.

2. Relax and repeat on your right leg. Repeat for a total of 10 stretches on each leg.

Exercise 5: DOUBLE LEG CIRCLES

To start: Lie on your back extending both legs into the air, keeping the pelvis stable, holding your belly button to your spine. Do not wiggle your hips.

Instructions:

1. Direct both legs simultaneously outward making a large circle returning to the starting position.

2. Repeat 10 times, then reverse the movement 10 times.

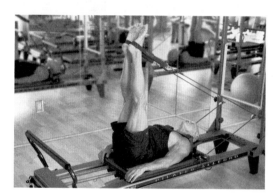 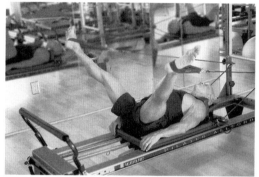

Exercise 6: ADDUCTOR STRETCH

To start: Sit on the floor with a Thera-Band or on the Reformer, opening both legs out to the side.

Instructions:

1. Hold the Thera-Band in both hands and wrap it around both feet.

2. Hold the stretch for a few seconds and then return to the starting position.

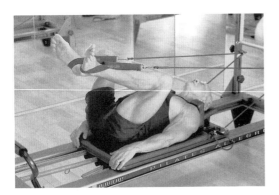 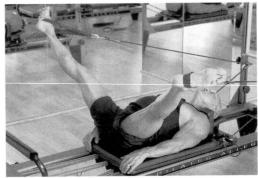

Exercise 7: IT BAND STRETCH

You should feel this stretch from your hip to your knee, along the side of your leg.

To start: Sit on the floor with a Thera-Band or on the Reformer.

Instructions:

1. Hold the Thera-Band with your right hand. Let your left knee fall in toward and across the midline of your body so your legs are crossing. This helps keep the pelvis balanced. Repeat with opposite leg positions.

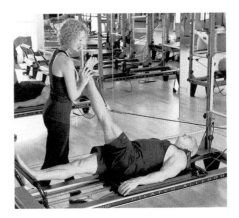

Exercise 8: FULL ROLL-UP

To start: Lie on your back with legs extended and arms over head.

Instructions:

1. Stretch over your legs reaching with your hands to your feet. Follow a sequence of arms, head, neck, shoulders, lifting and rolling up through the spine like a wheel. Exhale as you roll up.

2. Inhale and hold the stretch.

3. Exhale and roll your body back down. Start movement from the tailbone, rolling the spine down one vertebra down at a time. Pull your belly button to your backbone as you roll your body flat to the floor.

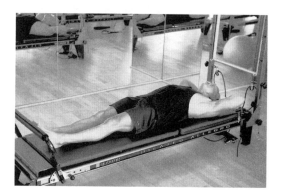 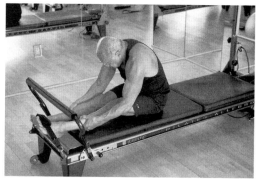

Exercise 9: SUPINE AB SERIES

To start: Lie on your back extending your legs straight into the air at a 90-degree angle to your hips. Hands are pointing up toward the ceiling, arms are straight.

Instructions:

1. Lower your arms from starting position to the floor and back up, curling your body up each time. Exhale as you roll up. Roll up to at least the bottom of your shoulder blades. Repeat 10 times.

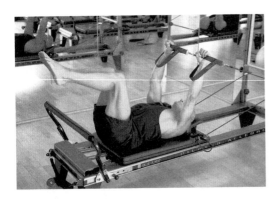 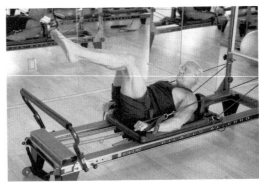

Exercise 10: SINGLE LEG EXTENSION FOR ABS

To start: Lie on the floor with the upper half of your legs perpendicular to the floor and the bottom half of your legs parallel to the floor. Hands are pointing up toward the ceiling, arms are straight.

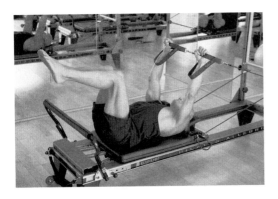 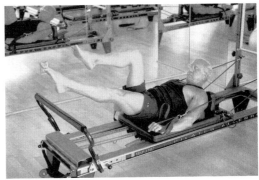

Instructions:

1. Extend your left leg out straight as your arms float down.

2. Bring your leg back as your arms float up to start position. Alternate sides 10 times with a flat back.

3. Next, add curling your body up with each leg extension. Exhale as you roll up. Roll up to at least the bottom of your shoulder blades. Repeat 10 times.

Exercise 11: DOUBLE LEG EXTENSION FOR ABS

To start: Lie on the floor with the upper half of your legs perpendicular to the floor and the bottom half of your legs parallel to the floor. This is called the "table top" position. Your arms are extended toward the ceiling.

Instructions:

1. Extend both legs out, keeping your back flat on the mat.

2. Pull legs back to table top as your arms float up. Repeat 10 times.

3. Add curling your body up with each leg extension. Exhale as you roll up. Roll up to at least the bottom of your shoulder blades. Repeat 10 times.

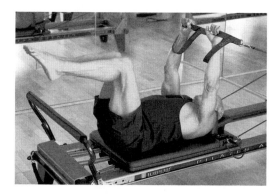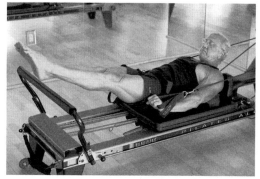

Exercise 12: BACK EXTENSIONS

To start: Lie on your stomach with hands behind your head and your legs extended back. You should be looking at the floor.

Instructions:

1. Lead the movement with your nose, as if you're rolling a marble with the tip of your nose, and lift your body up.

2. Roll your body back down to starting position. Repeat 10 times.

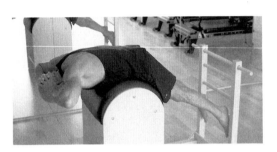
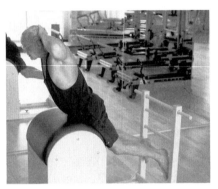

Exercise 13: LUNGES

To start: Standing tall, place your left foot in front of the right, extending your right leg back straight.

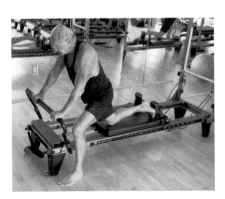
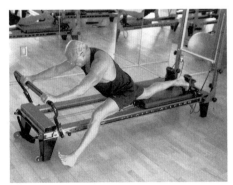

Instructions:

1. Bend your left knee so it is at a 90-degree angle with your knee above your ankle. Right leg reaches back away from your body. You should be actively pressing your hips to the floor.

2. Repeat with opposite leg.

The Life Plan Balance Workout

Improving your balance requires very little extra time out of your day. Balance training should be systematic, progressive, and functional, so begin with the exercises that fit your particular balance level, and work your way into the more advanced levels. You will be performing one of these exercises after your Pilates workout. There are three types of balance exercises, so mix them up as you see fit.

Test Your Ability to Balance

The first step to improving your balance is to determine your current balance level. The following are some tests you can do at home. If you already think your ability to balance is compromised, have someone close by watch you complete these. Time yourself to accurately document how long you are able to hold the position, and this will be your baseline—that is, your starting point. Then, test yourself once a week to see if you can hold these positions longer, which will indicate that you have better balance.

- Single leg reach—stand on one leg with your eyes opened or closed and extend your nonsupporting leg to the front, side, or back. Hold this position for as long as you can.

- Stork test—standing with your arms out to your side, bring the bottom of one foot to the inside knee of the other leg and hold that position with your eyes opened or closed for as long as you can.

On-the-Go Balance Training

The following is a list of simple ways to improve balance that you can do anytime, anywhere.

1. Walk through your house as if you were walking on a tightrope. Walk by placing the toe of one foot touching the heel of the other, then place the lagging foot at the toe of the front foot. Repeat until you reach your destination. You can also do this outside on a curb.

2. Figure 8 walking. Walk in a figure 8 progressively more quickly, with the 8 getting smaller and smaller.

3. Stand on one foot for 30-second intervals. A good goal is at least 60 seconds per foot. Keep track so you can see how you progress each month.

4. Balance on one leg while performing daily activities (brushing teeth, cooking, showering, and combing your hair). Remember to keep the knee slightly bent.

5. Pick up objects (newspaper, shoes, pen, and so on), while standing on one leg. This may not sound very hard, but be sure to have something nearby to hold on to just in case you fall.

Traditional Balance Exercises

STEP UP BALANCE

To start: Stand in front of a step or a level box with your feet shoulder width apart.

Instructions:

1. Step onto the step with your left leg.

2. Lift your right leg up until your upper leg is parallel to the floor.

3. Step down with both legs.

4. Repeat steps 1 and 2 for 10–20 repetitions, switching legs.

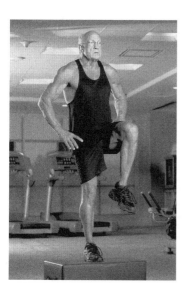 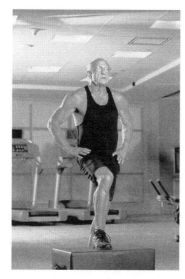

SINGLE LEG BALANCE

To start: Stand with your feet shoulder width apart. It's a good idea to perform this exercise near a wall in case you lose your balance.

Instructions:

1. Slowly lift one leg a minimum of 6 inches off the floor.

2. Hold this position for about 30 seconds.

3. Lower your leg to the floor and repeat 10–20 times, switching sides each time.

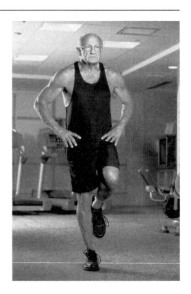

SINGLE LEG SQUAT

To start: Stand with your feet shoulder width apart. It's a good idea to perform this exercise near a wall in case you lose your balance.

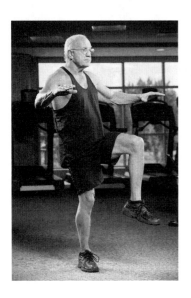
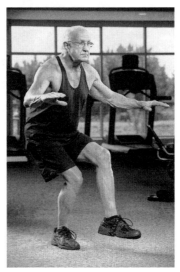

Instructions:

1. Lift one leg about 6 inches off the floor.

2. Lower your body to the floor by bending the knee of the planted leg and keeping the opposite leg off the floor.

3. Continue to squat down until the planted leg reaches a 45-degree angle.

4. Return to starting position and repeat 10–20 times with each leg.

SINGLE LEG TOE TOUCH

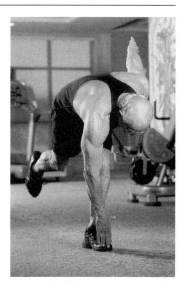

To start: Stand with your feet shoulder width apart. It's a good idea to perform this exercise near a wall in case you lose your balance.

Instructions:

1. Lift your right leg off the floor 6 inches.

2. Lean forward at the waist and touch your left foot with your right hand.

3. Return to starting position and repeat 10–20 times, switching legs each time.

Core/Abdominal Training

Most men think the core is synonymous with abdominal muscles. The "core" actually consists of many different muscles that stabilize the spine and pelvis and run the entire length of the torso. These muscles provide a solid foundation for movement of the extremities. Having a strong core is like building a strong foundation for a house. A house with a weak foundation cannot withstand the conditions that it has to face year to year. Similarly, if you have a weak core you will not be able to withstand the demands of day-to-day activities without pain, especially back pain. A weak core affects your overall fitness, athletic performance, and sexual performance.

On this program you will be performing core work following your balance exercise. Pick one each time from the following list.

PLANK

To start: Assume a modified pushup position, on your forearms and toes. Your body will form a straight line from your shoulders to your ankles.

Instructions:

1. Pull your abs in but don't stick out your butt.

2. Hold this position with a straight body for as long as you can. The goal is to work up to holding the plank for as long as 2 to 3 minutes.

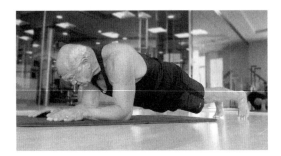

OPPOSITE ARM LEG REACH

To start: Position your body on a mat or floor in plank position.

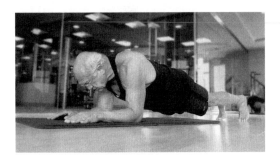 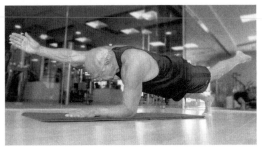

Instructions:

1. Extend one leg and the opposite arm so that they are parallel to the floor.

2. Hold this position for 3 to 4 seconds, and then repeat with the opposite arm and leg.

3. Begin with 10 reps on each side, ensuring that your back does not sag at any time.

SUPERMANS

To start: Lie facedown on the floor with your ankles extended and the tops of your toes on the ground.

Instructions:

1. Extend your arms on the floor out to your sides in a T position with your palms facing down.

2. Pressing your shoulder blades down and back, lift up your arms perpendicular to your body, forming a T shape. Hold this position for 30 to 60 seconds. Repeat 10 to 15 times.

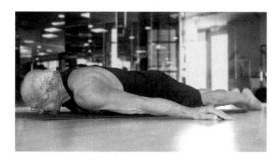 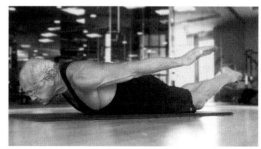

DR. LIFE'S SECRET AB STRETCH

My tightest muscles are my hamstrings, lower back, and abdominals. After my cardio workout I always spend 10–15 minutes stretching my hamstrings and lower back. Then I stretch my abdominals by lying on an exercise ball (or Ladder Barrel, as in the photo), on my back, and bending back as far as

I can. I hold this stretch for about 30–45 seconds and then repeat after a 15- to 30-second rest. I do 4 to 5 sets of this exercise. I believe it really has helped improve my posture and flatten my abdomen. It has also helped tighten my abdominal skin and accentuate my abs. I also do this exercise after my abdominal crunches: It's a perfect way to finish off my abs workout. Try it and you will be amazed at how it tightens and flattens your belly.

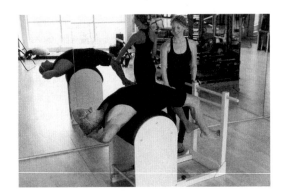

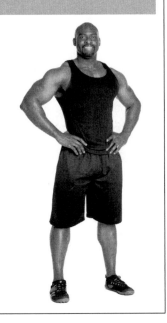

MEET ROD

Rod Stanley is my personal trainer and my friend. And just by looking at him, you can tell he's in great shape. Rod is 33 years old and has been working with me as my trainer for almost six years. Rod is a former Marine, a fitness therapist, and a nationally certified personal trainer: I work only with the best. But what you wouldn't know by looking at him is that he also spends a lot of time working on his flexibility and stretching.

"I've learned a lot from Dr. Life. He's taught me about internal health and the role that maintaining hormone levels plays in the role of healthy body composition, energy, and sexual function. He's also encouraged me to incorporate more flexibility and stretching into my own workouts, as well as the ones I create for my clients.

"Flexibility is absolutely necessary in order to perform any workout properly. If you're inflexible or have tight muscles it will make you prone to injuring yourself during your cardio and resistance-training workouts. It is also important when it comes to mastering weight-lifting technique.

"I know I'm nowhere near as old as Dr. Life, but even at 33 I find that I have to work more flexibility into my workouts as I'm getting older. Every day as I age I find that flexibility is more and more important, because overuse injuries or tightness can affect my workouts. Every day requires a little more attention than when I was younger. When I don't have time for a full hour Pilates class, I'll incorporate stretching into my resistance-training program. I may stretch an opposing muscle group: For example, after I do a bunch of chest exercises, during the rest period I'll stretch out my back muscles.

"When I first met Dr. Life I was in my late twenties. He initially called me because he wanted me to train him like I train myself. But he was 69! His goal was to do dumbbell chest presses with 100-pound dumbbells for a photo shoot. I couldn't believe it. But we did it, and he never complained. He shattered all my notions of what an old person should be doing, and now I use him as a motivational example for all my clients, even the ones in their forties or fifties who are moaning and groaning that they can't do the work because they are too old. I just point to Dr. Life, who at 74 still has the stamina and drive and works harder than over 90 percent of people I know. If he started at my age, he'd be stronger than me today.

"I also know that one of the main reasons that he's been able to keep his training up is that he incorporates so much flexibility into his workout. With proper flexibility he can avoid many injuries and avoid excessive stress on his joints, making him less prone to injury. It's absolutely key for him and all men to remain flexible so that they can continue to perform athletically at a high level."

• • •

I can't emphasize enough how important stretching is to maintaining an injury-free body as well as to sculpting the body that you want. You'll see in the next two chapters that stretching is a part of everything: You need to do it before your resistance-training workout (and after), and following your cardio work as well. Each of those workouts has its own stretching routine. But don't worry: Those stretching exercises won't take more than 10 minutes, tops.

In Chapter 8 you'll see how all of these workouts come together, so that you can schedule your entire week ahead of time, and know exactly what you'll be working on every day. But first, let's explore the Life Plan Resistance-Training Workout.

CHAPTER 6

The Life Plan Resistance-Training Workout

Y ou may be living proof that the human body loses muscle mass and gains body fat as it ages. This is what the so-called experts believe, but I know that it doesn't have to be this way. In fact, this is the last thing you want to have happen, because it is a surefire way to find yourself in a nursing home for the last years of your life.

While diet is critical for losing weight, I have found that regular, vigorous exercise is the only way to get rid of body fat and keep it off, while at the same time preventing muscle loss. And of all the modalities that you need to do, resistance training is by far the best way to teach your body to continuously burn calories. Resistance training, or weight-lifting, is how you are going to lose your excess body fat and achieve (and better still, maintain) a high level of strength, muscle mass, and physical fitness. I'm living proof that we can prove the experts wrong: You don't have to lose muscle mass and strength as you age, unless you let it happen!

Yet while many men are intrigued by resistance training, I find that they are fearful or hesitant. My patients are commonly concerned that they are going to hurt themselves, wrench their backs, or drop a weight and end up breaking their foot or something. My response to this is always the same: In the 15 years that I've been actively working out, I've never hurt myself lifting weights because I make sure I always warm up with lighter weights, use good form, and use weights that I can lift for at least six reps. And while I do get sore from time to time after a good workout, I never train to the point of physical pain. If I experience any pain during a workout I immediately stop the exercise.

Resistance training is the absolute key to my success. Correcting hormone deficiencies and cardio are important but without resistance training I would never look or feel as good as I do. This type of exercise generally involves lifting weights, but can be accomplished by using either all or part of your body weight as a resistance, or moving your body against some externally imposed resistance, such as elastic resistance bands, free weights, or strength-training machines. It can be performed anywhere: the local gym or your home, or even when you are on the road.

What Happens During Resistance Training?

During each strenuous workout, the microscopic fibers of your muscle tissues are torn or injured, which then forces your body to adapt by repairing this damaged tissue after your workout. This repair process makes your muscle bigger and stronger by adding more and larger muscle cells during the repair. Simply put, you tear down muscle during a workout, and then your body builds it back up again between workouts, making it bigger and stronger. The recovery period is critical to maximize growth and avoid overtraining and injury.

Resistance training can improve both muscular strength and endurance and helps you not only prevent muscle loss, but also creates new gains in muscle size and strength. After an intense workout, your body repairs the damaged muscle through a combination of sleep, the right kind of nutrition, and maintaining proper hormone levels. You also need to maintain your muscle- and strength-building program with persistence and consistency. It takes months to increase muscle mass, but it doesn't take much of an increase in muscle tissue to dramatically improve your strength, health, and appearance. Working with weights as light as five pounds can still make an enormous difference to your physique.

The best part is that building new muscle cells takes lots of energy, which is why building muscle burns calories. So not only are you getting bigger muscles, you're burning up body fat (providing you are on the correct nutrition program, one that will allow for fat loss, such as the Life Plan Diets). Train hard often enough, and your body will be conditioned to constantly burn more calories, day and night. And since all that repaired muscle is now bigger muscle—which takes more kilocalories to maintain—your metabolic rate increases. The more muscle you have, the more kilocalories you burn, even when you sleep, and the leaner you will get and stay—truly a win-win-win phenomenon!

Study after study has shown the importance of strength training in the prevention and rehabilitation of many chronic diseases, including osteoporosis, diabetes, depression, sarcopenia, lower-back pain, and heart disease. Aggressive resistance training is the first line of defense against sarcopenia—loss of muscle mass with aging, the number-one cause of nursing home admissions. Aging, degenerating, and dying mitochondria are now thought to play the key role in causing sarcopenia. Mitochondria are microscopic organelles that are found inside our cells, especially muscle cells. They are the principal sites where all of our energy is generated. As our mitochondria age they lose their ability to produce energy and muscle cells shrivel and die. If dying and degenerating mitochondria could be replaced with new, young, vibrant mitochondria, muscle and strength loss could be avoided. The good news is that we now know how to do this: Consistent, intense resistance training can induce adaptations that replace your old, dying mitochondria with brand-new mitochondria, no matter what your age is today. This is what the Life Plan is all about.

As muscle mass decreases, resting metabolic rate (RMR), muscle strength, and activity levels also decrease. As our RMR declines, our calorie requirements also decline. Most men, however, don't reduce their caloric intake, and their body fat begins to increase. This alone promotes many serious disease states, including insulin resistance and dyslipidemia (high cholesterol, low HDL, high triglycerides, and high LDL), which damage blood vessels and cause heart disease and heart attack, the number-one killer of American men.

Strength training also helps maintain and even increase bone density, further reducing the risk of fractures. In fact, high-intensity strength training is the only type of exercise that will prevent and actually treat osteoporosis and other degenerative bone disorders. Strength training decreases and in most cases alleviates back pain. While all forms of exercise have been shown to benefit men with chronic lower-back pain, an intense, integrated approach like the Life Plan has been proven to be the most effective. This strategy not only improves endurance and activity tolerance but also increases strength

START WITH A DOCTOR'S VISIT

It is critically important to see your doctor before you start a resistance-training program (or any exercise program for that matter), especially if you suffer frequently from back pain. Once you get the green light from your doctor, focus on exercises that strengthen the muscles that support your back, which include the abdominal and lower-back muscles. Be sure to conduct your exercises in a slow and controlled manner, and always use perfect form with each exercise.

and flexibility of your back muscles. In addition, it promotes weight loss (obesity is a major cause of acute and chronic back pain) and provides beneficial psychological effects.

DETERMINE YOUR 1-REP MAX

A phrase you'll hear often in the weight-training world is "1-rep max." This refers to the maximum weight you can use for a particular exercise if you were to only do it one time, that is, one rep. To determine your 1-rep max, use the calculators on my website (www.drlife.com). All you have to do is enter the amount of weight that you lifted and the number of reps you were able to perform and the calculator will estimate your 1-rep max. Choose a weight at which you can do no more than 10 reps to determine your 1-rep max.

In a 2009 study published in the *Archives of Physical Medicine and Rehabilitation*, Dr. B. W. Nelson and colleagues set out to determine if back-pain patients recommended for spinal surgery could avoid their surgery through an aggressive strengthening program. After following a 10-week intensive back-strengthening regimen, 57 of the 60 patients no longer required surgery and were virtually pain free.

Sore Muscles Mean You're Working Hard

It's normal to have some muscle pain after a good workout. In fact, this is usually an indication that you trained your muscles properly. You must achieve muscle soreness (often referred to as "good pain") after each training session. Good pain is soreness that is bilateral (both sides), not sharp or extreme, and lets you know that you worked your muscles just right. It's a great feeling.

Occasionally, you may feel pain that is excessive and that may even interfere with your training program. Ibuprofen, or another nonsteroidal anti-inflammatory drug, is frequently used to alleviate this kind of pain, but these medications can interfere with your muscle repair and growth processes. I never take them for this kind of muscle discomfort. I basically do my best to ignore it. I don't like to cover it up. I want to know what's going on, and pain meds prevent this by masking my pain. Instead, I take my vitamins, fish oil, and other supplements, which reduce inflammation and speed up the recovery process naturally.

Scientists believe the muscle pain associated with intense exercise is caused, in part, by the excessive production of free radicals during exercise. Free radicals help repair the microscopic tears and inflammation we want to produce in our muscle tissue when we train hard, and they actually promote increases in strength and growth. Excessive amounts of these molecules, however, can actually do more harm than good and interfere with muscle healing. We have known for some time now that antioxidants including vitamin E, vitamin C, and selenium help neutralize free-radical activity. They may also help prevent the excessive muscle damage from free radicals that intense exercise can cause. So, train hard, take your antioxidants, eat healthy, and enjoy the "good" pain you get in your muscles after a great workout that lets you know you are doing it right and making progress.

TRAIN LIKE YOUR LIFE DEPENDS ON IT—BECAUSE IT DOES

Health is much more than the absence of disease—I define it as mental clarity that accompanies strength plus energy. Many aspects of the Life Plan will give you more energy, but only resistance training can increase your strength. This is important because increased strength can improve all areas of your life:

- Enables men to have a more powerful presence
- Enhances self-confidence
- Protects the body from the hard spills that often accompany aging

Resistance Training 101

The components of a good resistance-training program include strengthening every muscle group in your body: legs, arms, back, chest, shoulders, and core. Training of all these muscle groups is done by completing various exercises at a particular frequency (how many times you work a muscle group in a set time frame, i.e. reps), duration (how long you take to complete a set workout pose), and intensity (percentage of 1-rep max you use for a particular exercise).

You will need to follow this resistance-training program five days per week to achieve the best results. It is very important to train your whole body in a way that stresses every muscle during each workout, and over the course of the week you'll do just that. You cannot do resistance training on the same set of muscles every day because your muscle tissues need time and rest to recover from each training session in order to grow. If you trained every day, you would only be breaking down the muscle, and not letting it repair. Worse, the body will respond to overtraining by actually decreasing strength, mass, and performance.

A full-body weekly routine is more advantageous in this beginner's phase because your goal is not to increase muscle size and strength, but to train your nervous system to interact with your muscular system. By doing so, you will also be burning more calories. Training the whole body, particularly a circuit workout, causes the heart to work harder to pump blood and oxygen to the muscles that are performing the work. This results in higher heart rate, which equates to a higher caloric expenditure.

The danger of not training the whole body in a balanced way is that you set yourself up for muscular imbalances, postural distortions, and interference with reciprocal inhibition (when muscles on the opposite sides of a joint contract at the same time, producing muscle tears). This causes undue stress on the joints and soft tissues of your body. All that just means one word: injury. Injuries can set you back months and, in some cases, years. Avoid injuries at all costs. Move slowly through your exercise journey. This is a lifetime approach to fitness, not a 12-week race to meet your goals.

You should continue with this phase for four to six weeks before you can assess your results. And once you master these exercises and are ready for a more intense workout afterward, follow the programs in *The Life Plan*.

Your resistance-training workout will contain these core components:

- Warmup

- Stretching

- Exercise

- Cooldown

The Warmup

Before you begin resistance training it is important to prepare your body mentally and physically to exercise. Warming up is the first critical step because it improves your performance significantly. When your muscles are warmed up they will contract more forcefully and relax more quickly, which decreases the risk of overstretching or overstressing your muscles. This is the key to avoiding injuries.

A warmup in this case is a very brief cardio interval: It could be walking on a treadmill, riding a stationary or street bike, or running for three to five minutes, followed by a couple of light sets of your first strength-training exercise. The Life Plan Workout is designed with a warmup built in. If you follow the workout as it is outlined in Chapter 8, you will not need to do an additional warmup. However, if you want to add an additional resistance-training workout to your week, then you must warm up first.

Stretching Out with SMR

Stretching helps avoid injury and improves overall performance. A brief set of self myofascial release (SMR) can be done before resistance training and after your brief cardio warmup if you have excessive muscle. The fascia is the soft portion of the connective tissues and provides support for most tissues in the body, including the muscles. This soft tissue can become restricted due to trauma, injury, overuse, or inactivity, causing pain and tension. It can also limit the ability of the muscles to have proper blood flow. As in most tissue, irritation causes localized inflammation, which also leads to pain. Worse, chronic inflammation results in fibrosis, or the thickening of the connective tissue, and results in reflexive muscle tension that causes even more pain and inflammation. Myofascial techniques aim to break this cycle for your legs and back muscles.

The technique I use for myofascial release is called "foam rolling" and requires that you purchase a foam roller at any sporting goods store, or on the Internet. Most gyms also have these on hand.

Place the foam roller under each muscle group until a tender area is found, and maintain pressure on the tender area for 30–60 seconds. This will result in releasing the fascia, and softening and lengthening the muscle. It will help break down scar tissue and allow the muscles to reach optimal levels of lengthening during exercise. In less than 10 minutes, you'll be completely stretched and ready for resistance training.

AREAS FOR FOAM ROLLING:

- Inner thigh
- Calves
- Back (upper)
- Quadriceps
- Outer leg (lying on side)
- Hamstring
- Peroneals (lower leg)
- Midback
- Gluteus

PREVENTING LEG CRAMPS

Near the end of a hard set of hamstring curls, you may feel a cramp starting to come on and find that you have to stop the set. These cramps are usually a result of poor conditioning, sluggish blood flow to the muscles, dehydration, and poor flexibility. Flexibility is a very important aspect of our total conditioning. Tight muscles get much less blood circulating through them than relaxed muscles. In a flexible person, blood moves freely and unimpeded through their exercising muscles, flushing out lactic acid and providing vital oxygen to muscle cells. It is this lack of oxygen combined with high levels of lactic acid that can cause pain and cramping.

When you include stretching exercises before resistance training you can prevent cramping and delay the development of fatigue. If your hamstrings cramp up like mine used to, just massage the muscle, stretch it out, and get back to work. As your strength, conditioning, and flexibility improve these cramps will become a thing of the past.

The Reps

Each of the exercises below is measured in repetitions and sets. A repetition is one complete movement of a particular exercise. There are three phases of a repetition:

1. Eccentric contraction—the negative portion of the lift where the muscle lengthens to slow down the force (for example, in a bench press exercise when you bring the barbell down toward your chest). The contraction occurs when you are resisting the pull of gravity by not allowing the weight to fall on your chest.

2. Isometric contraction of the muscle—the top or bottom portion of the lift when the muscle is static and the force is not being moved at all.

3. Concentric contraction—the positive portion of the lift where the muscle shortens to exert force against the weight (for example, when you push the barbell up), that is, against gravity.

The speed—or tempo— at which you perform a repetition is determined by your fitness goals. If you have not been working out consistently in the past, it's important to increase your muscular endurance before you develop increased strength. The workout that follows is built around a tempo perfect for increasing endurance. Once you've mastered this, you can continue with the more strength-oriented programs in *The Life Plan*.

The Set

A number of repetitions performed one after another make up a set. The general rule is it takes between 400 and 500 reps of a particular exercise to train your body to perform it correctly. You shouldn't train to muscle failure until your body has reached the point of total comfort with the exercise. Once you've got the form down pat and your nervous system, joints, and muscle stabilizers are strong enough to keep the weight steady, you can then go to muscle failure. At that point, you can also branch out into other types of training if desired, such as strength training, where the optimal rep range is six to eight repetitions and three to four sets.

The Rest Period

Between sets, you should take a rest break. The rest period for an endurance workout between sets is usually 30–60 seconds; in strength training, two to three minutes.

Intensity

Intensity refers to the amount of force you should use—that is, how heavy the weight should be. Endurance training uses an intensity of 50 to 70 percent of your 1-rep max (again, each repetition should be at a weight equal to 50 to 70 percent of the maximum amount of weight you can lift on that particular exercise if you were to do it only one time). Strength training uses 75 to 85 percent of your 1-rep max.

The Cooldown

Each session should end with a cooldown period such as walking/running on the treadmill or getting on the stationary bike for five minutes at about 45 to 50 percent of your target heart rate to bring your body back to a resting state. The stretching program in Chapter 5 is an excellent way to cool down if you have the time. The Life Plan Workout is designed with a cooldown built in. If you follow the workout as it is designed in Chapter 8, you will not need to do an additional cooldown. However, if you want to add an additional resistance-training workout to your week, then you must add a cooldown when you are done.

Lift Weights Now, Enjoy Sex Later

Lifting heavy weights and performing compound movements (squats, deadlifts, and bench presses) increases serum testosterone and growth hormone levels—key hormones to improve sexual function.

The Life Plan Resistance Gym Workout

The following chart shows the exact routine I follow every day. Unless you have a full equipment setup sitting in your basement, you'll need to do these exercises at the gym. Do these exercises as listed below, and do not skip any of them. Use the accompanying photos to guide you toward proper alignment and posture. You can also work with a trainer and follow the program together so that he or she can make sure you are in the right position every time. Completing this routine will take about one hour. I do this first thing in the morning, but any time is fine, as long as it works for you and you don't miss workouts.

You will start with 2–3 sets per exercise, 15–25 repetitions, and 45- to 90-second rest periods. Each rep should be performed at a slow pace of around 8 seconds each.

For example, each of the suggested exercises will look like this: Dumbbell Lateral Raise—5 lb, 2–3 sets of 15–25 repetitions, 45–90 seconds rest after each set.

The purpose of the higher repetitions and short rest periods is to build your muscular endurance as well as increase the integrity of the joints and connective tissues. Beginners do not possess high levels of neuromuscular control, so it's important to perform your sets with lighter weights to help increase your ability to stabilize the weights. Do not rush the speed of the repetitions. Perform all repetitions at the tempo, or speed, in seconds, as listed below (4 seconds eccentric, 1 second isometric, 2 seconds concentric).

MONDAY EXERCISE	Sets	Reps	Intensity	Rest	Tempo
Warm up 5 min					
ABS					
Ab machine	4	12–15	80%–90%	90–120 sec	2-2-2
CHEST					
DB chest press	4	8–12	80%–90%	90–120 sec	2-2-1
Machine press	4	8–12	80%–90%	90–120 sec	2-2-1
Incline DB press	4	8–12	80%–90%	90–120 sec	2-2-1
Machine fly	4	8–12	80%–90%	90–120 sec	2-2-1
COOL DOWN					

TUESDAY EXERCISE	Sets	Reps	Intensity	Rest	Tempo
Warm up 5 min					
BACK					
Machine row	4	8–12	80%–90%	90–120 sec	2-2-1
Lat pulldown	4	8–12	80%–90%	90–120 sec	2-2-1
Seated row	4	8–12	80%–90%	90–120 sec	2-2-1
Pull-ups	4	8–12	80%–90%	90–120 sec	2-2-1
COOL DOWN					

WEDNESDAY EXERCISE	Sets	Reps	Intensity	Rest	Tempo
Warm up 5 min					
ABS					
Ab machine	4	12–15	80%–90%	90–120 sec	2-2-2
LEGS					
Leg press	4	8–12	80%–90%	90–120 sec	2-2-1
Barbell squats	4	8–12	80%–90%	90–120 sec	2-2-1

WEDNESDAY EXERCISE	Sets	Reps	Intensity	Rest	Tempo
Leg ext	4	8–12	80%–90%	90–120 sec	2-2-1
Seated leg curl	4	8–12	80%–90%	90–120 sec	2-2-1

COOL DOWN

THURSDAY EXERCISE	Sets	Reps	Intensity	Rest	Tempo
Warm up 5 min					

SHOULDERS

	Sets	Reps	Intensity	Rest	Tempo
Overhead DB press	4	8–12	80%–90%	90–120 sec	2-2-1
Machine overhead press	4	8–12	80%–90%	90–120 sec	2-2-1
DB lateral raises	4	8–12	80%–90%	90–120 sec	2-2-1
Reverse fly	4	8–12	80%–90%	90–120 sec	2-2-1

COOL DOWN

FRIDAY EXERCISE	Sets	Reps	Intensity	Rest	Tempo
Warm up 5 min					

ABS

	Sets	Reps	Intensity	Rest	Tempo
Ab machine	4	12–15	80%–90%	90–120 sec	2-2-2

BICEPS

	Sets	Reps	Intensity	Rest	Tempo
Preacher curl	4	8–12	80%–90%	90–120 sec	2-2-1
Dumbbell curl	4	8–12	80%–90%	90–120 sec	2-2-1
EZ curl bar	4	8–12	80%–90%	90–120 sec	2-2-1

TRICEPS

	Sets	Reps	Intensity	Rest	Tempo
DB overhead ext	4	8–12	80%–90%	90–120 sec	2-2-1
Weighted dips	4	8–12	80%–90%	90–120 sec	2-2-1
Pushdowns	4	8–12	80%–90%	90–120 sec	2-2-1

COOL DOWN

At the Gym Exercise Descriptions

Chest

DUMBBELL BENCH CHEST PRESS

To start: Lie on your back on a flat bench. Hold a dumbbell in each hand on either side of your chest. Pull your navel inward.

1. Lifting both weights at the same pace, push them straight up toward the ceiling until your arms are fully extended.

2. Slowly lower the dumbbells and stop when your upper arms (triceps) are parallel to the floor.

3. Hold them there for 1 second, and then return to the starting position.

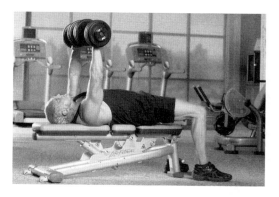 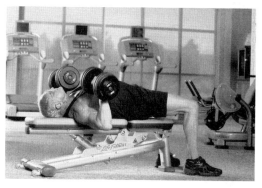

MACHINE CHEST PRESS

To start: Sit on the seated press machine, with your back firmly against the pad, your feet flat on the floor. Draw your navel inward. Adjust the seat so that machine handles are in line with your upper chest. Grasp the handles with a palms-down grip.

Instructions:

1. Push against the machine handles and extend your arm in front of you, contracting your chest muscles. Hold for 2 seconds.

2. Slowly lower the handles back to the starting position without letting the weight stack touch. Stop when your arms form a 90-degree angle.

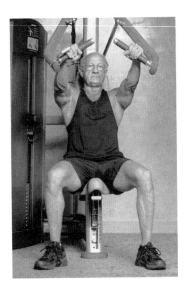 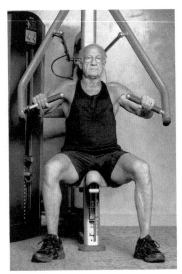

INCLINE DUMBBELL BENCH PRESS

To start: Lie on an incline bench set at approximately a 30- to 45-degreee angle. Keep your feet flat on the floor and draw your navel inward. Grab a pair of dumbbells, with a palms-down grip.

Instructions:

1. Extend your arms fully so the dumbbells are directly above your chest, almost touching each other. Pinch your shoulder blades against the pad.

2. Slowly lower the dumbbell to shoulder level. Your elbows should form a 90-degree angle.

3. Press the dumbbells upward, using your pectoral muscles. Straighten your arms fully and squeeze at the top.

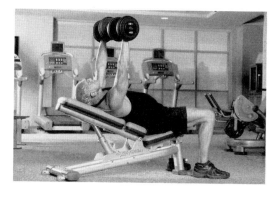
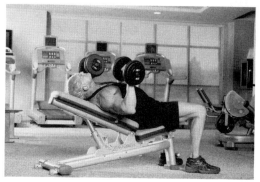

DECLINE DUMBBELL BENCH PRESS

To start: Lie on a decline bench with your feet anchored under the foot pad. Have someone hand you a pair of dumbbells and grab them with a palms-down grip.

Instructions:

1. Extend your arms fully so the dumbbells are directly above your chest, almost touching each other. Pinch your shoulder blades against the pad.

2. Slowly lower the dumbbell to shoulder level. Your elbows should form a 90-degree angle.

3. Press the dumbbells upward, using your pectoral muscles. Straighten your arms fully and squeeze at the top.

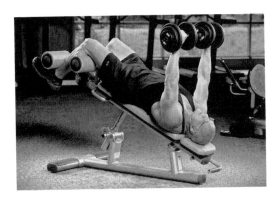 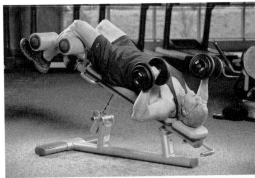

MACHINE FLY

To start: Adjust the seat of the machine so that your arms are in line with your shoulders. Sit with your torso erect against the back pad. Grasp the handles with your palms facing each other. Draw your navel inward.

Instructions:

1. Push the handles toward each other like you are hugging a large tree and contract your chest muscles hard at the end of the movement.

2. Slowly return your arms to the start position until your elbows are in line with your shoulders.

NOTE: Make sure your shoulders maintain full contact with the back pad.

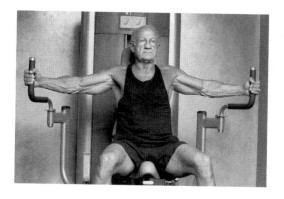 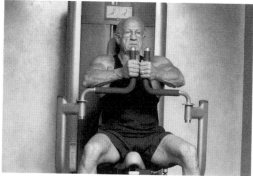

LAT PULLDOWN

To start: Sit at the lat pulldown machine. Adjust the knee pads so that they fit snugly over your thighs. Place your feet flat on the floor. Draw your navel inward. Keep your torso erect. Grasp the bar with your palms facing away from your body.

Instructions:

1. Draw your shoulder blades together and pull the bar down toward your chest, just past your chin.

2. Hold this position for 2 seconds.

3. Slowly straighten your arms, bringing the bar overhead.

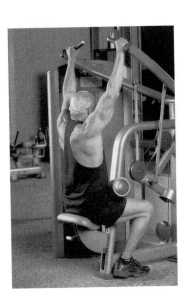 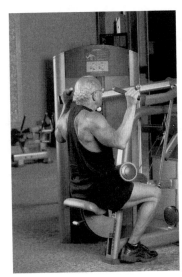

SEATED ROW

To start: Sit down at the base of a pulley machine. Draw your navel inward. Keep your back straight. Place your feet against the platform with your legs slightly bent. Choose a handle that has a double neutral grip (palms facing inward) and attach to the lower pulley cable.

Instructions:

1. Hold the handles and pull them toward your midsection.

2. Pull your shoulder blades together and contract your back muscles.

3. Extend your arms in front of you. Stop before your shoulder blades roll forward.

NOTE: Be sure to keep your torso erect.

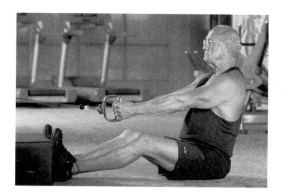 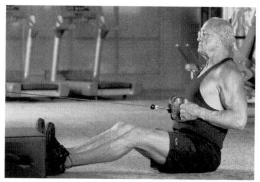

PULLUPS

To start: Grab the overhead bar with your palms facing away from your body slightly wider than shoulder width apart. Extend your arms and relax your shoulders to fully stretch your back. Draw your navel inward.

Instructions:

1. Pull yourself up until your chin is even with the bar.

2. Contract your back at the top of the movement.

3. Slowly lower to the starting position.

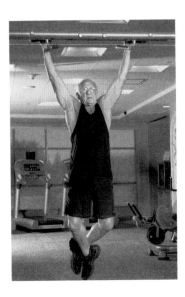 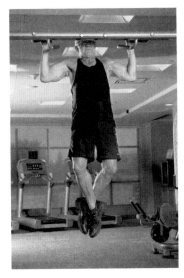

BARBELL ROW

To start: Stand upright, holding a barbell with palms facing inward. Keep your back straight and bend forward at the waist. Draw your navel inward. Keep your knees slightly bent. Extend your arms straight down.

Instructions:

1. Pull the barbell toward your lower rib cage. Concentrate on pulling with your back muscles.

2. Raise your elbows as high as possible.

3. Slowly lower your arms, returning to the starting position.

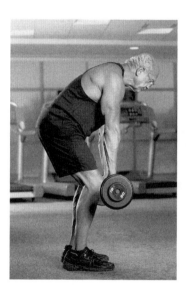 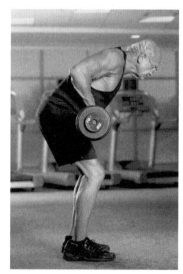

DUMBBELL ROW

To start: Kneel on a bench as pictured, holding a dumbbell in one hand.

Instructions:

1. Hinge yourself at the hips without losing the natural curve in your back. Your back should be almost parallel to the floor.

2. Bring the weight toward your chest by bending your elbows and squeezing your shoulder blades together without shrugging your shoulders. Return to the starting position.

3. Repeat with other hand.

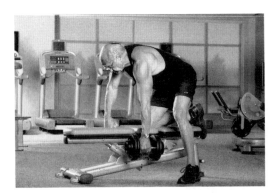 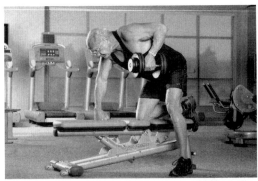

OVERHEAD DUMBBELL PRESS

To start: Sitting on the end of a bench, or on a seated bench apparatus, bring two dumbbells to shoulder height.

Instructions:

1. Press the weights directly overhead in an upside-down V pattern until they are touching each other and your arms are fully extended.

2. Then return to the starting position with upper arms (triceps) parallel to the floor.

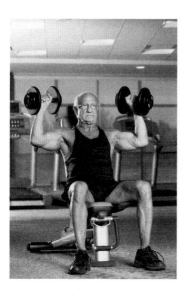 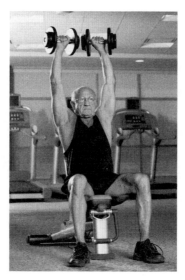

MACHINE OVERHEAD PRESS

To start: Adjust the seat to the proper height so that your upper arms are parallel to the floor. Sit on the machine with hands fixed on the bar and palms facing outward.

Instructions:

1. Press the bars upward until arms are fully extended; stop before arms are locked out.

2. Lower the machine until upper arms are parallel to the floor and arms make a 90-degree angle.

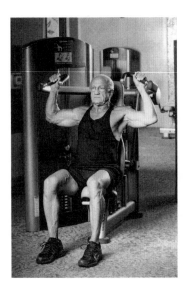 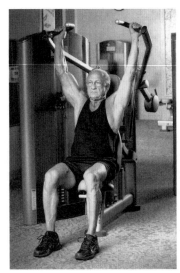

DUMBBELL LATERAL RAISE

To start: Stand erect with your feet closer than shoulder width apart, draw your navel inward. Grab a pair of 5- to 10-pound dumbbells with a palms-down grip.

Instructions:

1. Extend your arms out to your sides to shoulder level. Keep your elbows bent to a slightly greater than 90-degree angle. Hold for 2 seconds.

2. Slowly lower to the starting position.

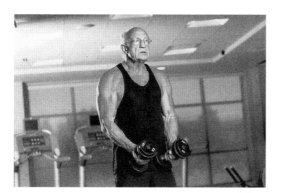 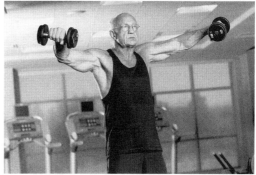

REVERSE FLY

To start: Sit on the end of a bench placing your feet firmly on the floor. Grab a dumbbell in each hand, draw your navel inward, and lean forward as far as possible.

Instructions:

1. Begin by placing your arms to your sides.

2. Contract your shoulder and back muscles as you bring the dumbbells to a horizontal position.

3. Slowly return to the starting position.

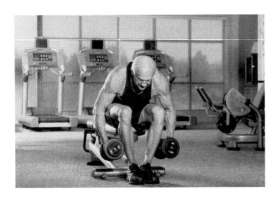 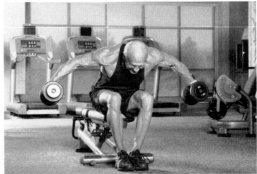

BARBELL SQUATS

To start: Stand inside a squat rack, with a barbell placed on the back of your neck. Grab the bar with a grip around 8 inches wider than shoulder width apart. Make sure the squat rack is equipped with safety bars.

Instructions:

1. Lower your body until the upper part of your leg is close to being parallel to the floor.

2. Keep chest up high throughout the motion.

3. Return to starting position by pressing upward, with the force mostly coming from the middle and heel portion of your feet.

4. Stop just before you lock your knees.

5. Repeat for the desired number of repetitions.

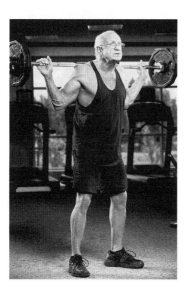 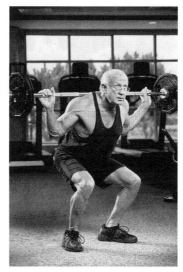

LEG PRESS

To start: Place your feet shoulder width apart on the platform of a leg press machine, turning them slightly outward. Unlock any safety devices and allow the weight to lower toward your chest.

Instructions:

1. Lower the weight until your legs form a 90-degree angle.

2. Drive into the platform, pressing through your heels and keeping your feet flat until your knees are almost fully extended.

3. Avoid locking out any joints while performing this exercise. Return to the starting position.

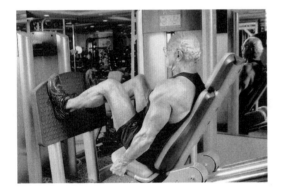 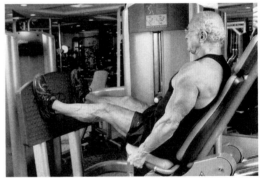

LEG EXTENSIONS

To start: Sit on the leg-extension machine seat with your back firmly pressed against the pad. Draw your navel inward. Adjust the rollers so that they press against your lower shins. Keep your feet flexed. Grasp the handles alongside the seat.

Instructions:

1. Straighten your legs slowly to their full extension and hold for 2 seconds. Do not lock your knees.

2. Lower them to the starting position.

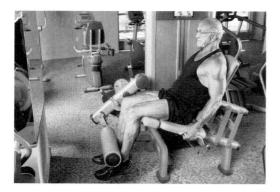 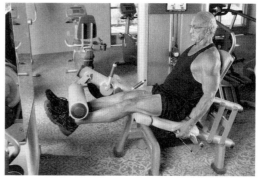

SEATED LEG CURLS

To start: Sit down on the leg curl machine with back firmly placed against the pad. Adjust the machine so the knee joint is in line with the pivot point on the machine. Place the back of your lower leg against padded lever and adjust the lap pad to fit firmly above your knees.

Instructions:

1. Pull lever to back of thighs by contracting hamstrings and flexing knees.

2. Return lever to staring position by extending the legs. Repeat. Make sure that you do not excessively arch back or allow body to slide down in the seat.

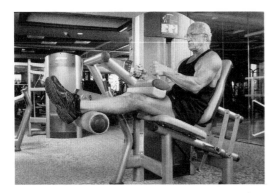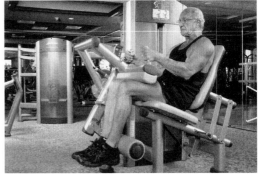

PREACHER CURL

To start: Stand at the Preacher Curl Machine. Place the back of your upper arm against the incline support pad. Maintain an erect position. Draw your navel inward.

Instructions:

1. With your upper arm firmly against the pad, grab the handles on the bar, curling your arms up toward your face.

2. Squeeze your biceps at the top of the movement.

3. Slowly lower to the starting position.

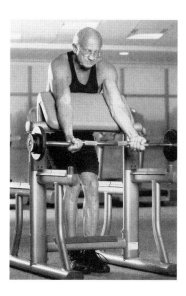
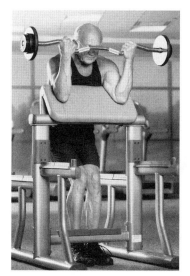

DUMBBELL CURL

To start: Sit in a chair holding two dumbbells at your side, with your palms facing your legs.

Instructions:

1. Curl the weights up by flexing your forearms toward your shoulders and your hands outward so that your palms are facing your shoulders when you reach the top.

2. Squeeze your biceps at the top of the movement.

3. Lower the dumbbells slowly to the starting posting.

4. Repeat for the prescribed number of reps.

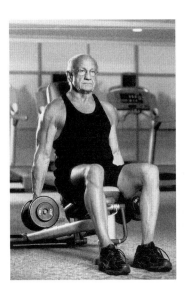 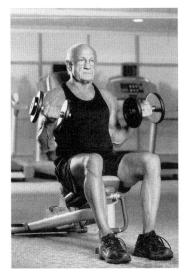

BARBELL CURL

To start: Stand with your feet shoulder width apart. Pull your navel inward. Hold a barbell with both hands at about shoulder width with a palms-up grip. Extend your arms in front of your thighs. Keep your elbows along the sides of your body.

Instructions:

1. Curl the barbell up toward your chest in a slow, controlled motion, contracting your biceps at the top, and hold contraction for 2 seconds.

2. Lower the bar slowly. Do not allow the bar to rest on your thighs.

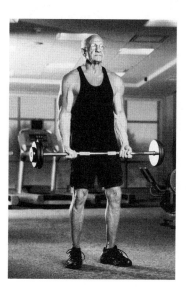 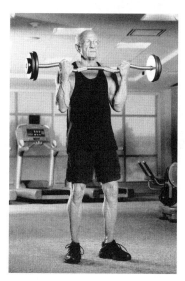

MACHINE CURL

To start: Sit in the chair and grab both handles firmly.

Instructions:

1. Curl the handles upward with your triceps firmly supported against the machine pads.

2. Squeeze your biceps at the top of the movement and hold contraction for 2 seconds.

3. Slowly return to the starting position.

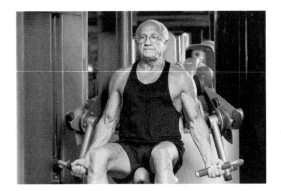
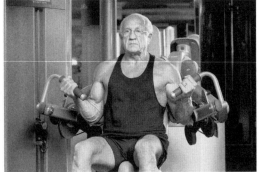

TRICEPS PUSHDOWN

To start: Stand in front of a high cable machine with your feet shoulder width apart. Draw your navel inward. Hook a V bar attachment and grab it with a palms-down grip. Keep your elbows at your sides.

Instructions:

1. Press the V bar down with your hands.

2. As you pass the 90-degree elbow position, straighten your arms out and squeeze your triceps hard and hold contraction for 2 seconds.

3. Slowly bring the V bar back up toward your chest. Stop when your upper arm is parallel to the floor.

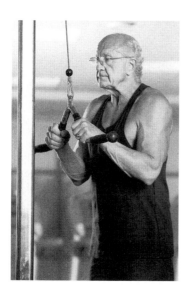 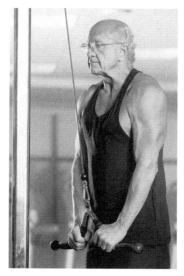

DUMBBELL OVERHEAD EXTENSION

To start: Sit on the edge of a chair with your feet flat on the floor, back straight and supported; with both hands, grab a dumbbell. Pull your navel inward.

Instructions:

1. Bend your elbow and raise your arms overhead. Keep your arms close to your ears and the dumbbells behind your head.

2. Keeping your upper arms stationary, lower the dumbbell behind your head until your elbows form a 90-degree angle.

3. Press the dumbbell upward until your arms are fully extended, and contract your triceps.

4. Repeat for the required number of repetitions.

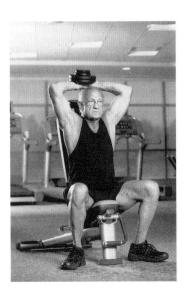 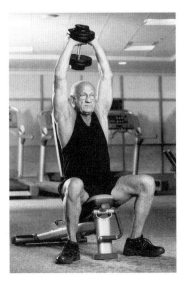

WEIGHTED DIPS

To start: You can use either a dip machine or parallel bars. Grasp the bars with a tight grip. Make sure you keep your chest up high. Bend your legs and look forward.

Instructions:

1. Begin with elbows extended while holding your body in the air.

2. In a controlled manner, lower your body by bending your elbows.

3. Continue lowering your body until your upper arms are parallel to the floor.

4. Push your body upward to the starting position by using your triceps, shoulders, and chest.

5. Stop just before you lock your elbows.

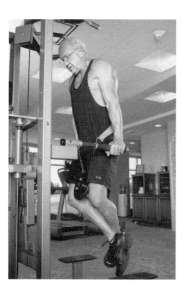 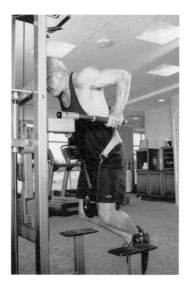

AB MACHINE

To start: Sit on the seat with your hands gripping the supports on both sides of your head and your feet pressed firmly on the floor or against the padded bar support if provided.

Instructions:

1. Keeping your back flat against the backrest, begin moving your elbows down, driving your lower rib cage toward your pelvis.

2. Slowly reverse the movement and repeat.

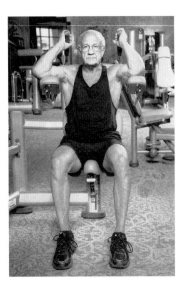 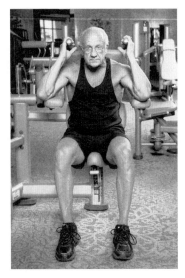

The Life Plan Resistance Home/Travel Workout

If you want to replicate what I do in the privacy of your home, on the road, or whenever you can't get to a gym, follow the routine as outlined below. This routine is different from the one above because it uses resistance bands and core floor exercises—the same ones you can use for the Pilates workout in Chapter 5. As you get stronger, you may need to replace older bands with newer ones with more resistance. Make sure you start with a band that allows you to experience muscle failure, or feel challenged, during each set.

The fact that you won't be "lifting" weights doesn't make your workout any less effective. As I've said, it's not the actual weight that matters, but all the factors that go into each repetition. When you use resistance bands you are working against your own body's weight and the band tension. So take these exercises just as seriously as you would if you were doing them at the gym, and I can guarantee that you will see results. Don't forget the warmup and the cooldown, and follow the total-body routine exactly as it is listed below.

You might find it more motivating to do these exercises in front of a mirror. Follow the directions carefully and use the photos to master each pose. Before you begin, make sure to do your SMR stretching for 5 to 10 minutes.

For each exercise you'll do 3 sets of 15 to 20 repetitions. Rest for 60 to 90 seconds between sets, and follow at a 2-2-2 tempo. Because this is a limited workout, you'll be doing a total-body workout each time. You can do this entire workout every other day, with a day of rest in between for best results.

PLANK OPPOSITE-ARM-LEG REACH

To start: Assume a modified pushup position, on your elbows and toes. Your body will form a straight line from your shoulders to your ankles. Pull your abs in but don't stick out your butt.

Instructions:

1. Extend your right arm straight in front of you until your arm is completely straight.

2. Lift your left leg off the floor about 5 inches. Hold for the allotted time.

3. Return to your original position and repeat with your left hand and right leg for the allotted time.

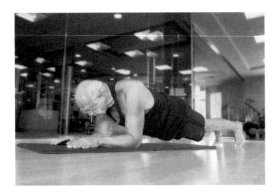 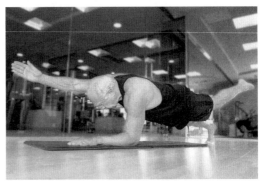

ABDOMINAL CRUNCH

To start: Lie with your back pressing against the floor. Place your hands loosely behind your head, knees bent, feet flat on the floor. Do not pull on your neck. Look up to the ceiling. Imagine that you have placed a tennis ball underneath your chin.

Instructions:

1. Begin to curl your upper body 2 inches off the floor.

2. Contract your abdominal muscles on the way up by bringing your rib cage toward your pelvis. Do not let your shoulder blades touch the floor.

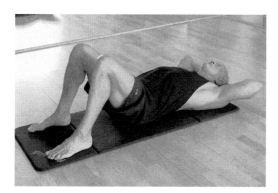 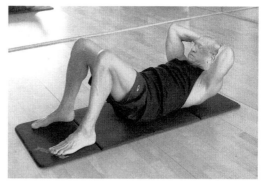

QUADRUPED OPPOSITE-ARM-LEG REACH

To start: Position your body on a mat or floor in all-fours position.

Instructions:

1. Extend one leg and the opposite arm so that they are parallel to the floor.

2. Hold this position for 3 to 4 seconds, and then repeat with the opposite arm and leg.

3. Perform prescribed number of reps on each side, ensuring that your back does not sag at any time.

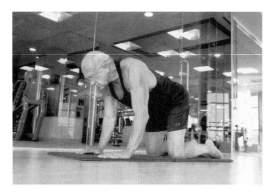
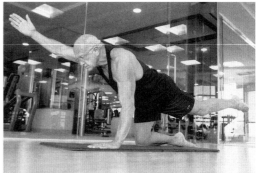

BICYCLE CRUNCH

To start: Lie on the floor with your hands loosely behind your head. Raise your legs to form a 90-degree angle at your knees.

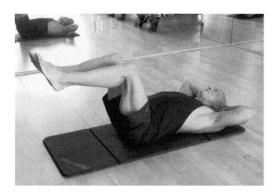
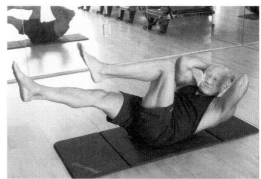

Instructions:

1. As you curl your upper body and crunch your abdominal muscles, bring your left elbow toward your right side while drawing your right knee in to meet it.

2. Continue rapidly to alternate sides.

RESISTANCE BAND CRUNCHES

To start: Sit in a chair and wrap the band around the underneath side of the chair. Run each part of the band up your back and firmly grasp the handles.

Instructions:

1. Contract your abdominal muscles as you move your lower rib cage toward your pelvis.

2. Hold the crunch position for 1 or 2 seconds.

3. Slowly return to the upright position.

4. Perform 15 to 25 reps and you will get a burn in your abs that will let you know you are making great progress.

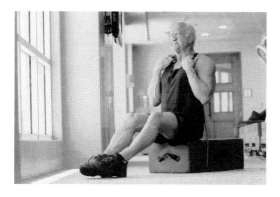 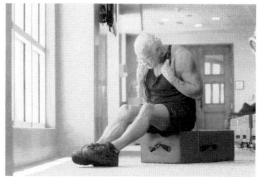

RESISTANCE BAND ONE-ARM FLIES

To start: Attach the band to a sturdy object at about shoulder height (standing or sitting), such as a piece of furniture or a closed door. Hold the handle in right hand and wrap the loop around your hand to increase tension if needed.

Instructions:

1. Keeping arms straight (elbow slightly bent) at shoulder level, contract the chest to bring the arm in toward the midchest. Return to start and repeat.

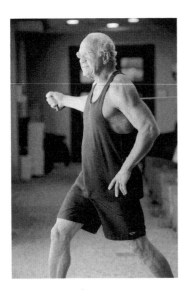 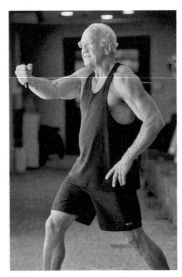

RESISTANCE BAND PUSHUPS

To start: Position yourself on your knees or toes and wrap the band over your back, holding on to the ends with both hands flat on the floor.

Instructions:

1. Loop the band to add tension, extend the legs to a straightened position, and bend elbows into a pushup. Return to starting position with arms extended, stopping before you lock the elbow.

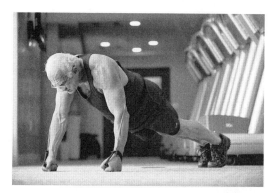 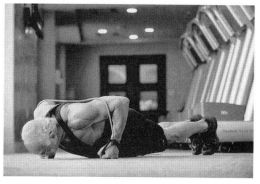

RESISTANCE BAND LAT PULLS

To start: Begin in a seated, kneeling, or standing position with your arms straight up overhead, holding the band toward the middle. Adjust hands closer to increase tension.

Instructions:

1. Contract your back and pull the band down while bringing the elbows toward the rib cage. Raise back up and repeat.

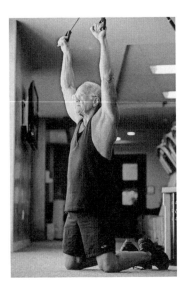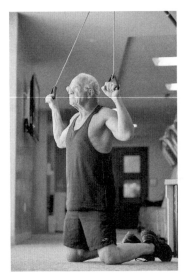

RESISTANCE BAND REAR DELT FLY

To start: Standing or sitting, hold band at chest level, arms straight out in front of you, hands a few inches apart.

Instructions:

1. Squeeze the shoulder blades together and pull band so that arms move out to the sides like an airplane.

2. Return to start and repeat, keeping tension on the band the entire time.

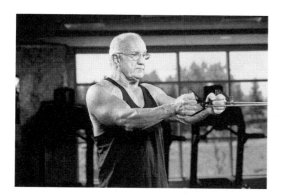 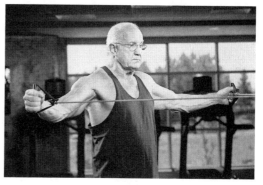

RESISTANCE BAND ONE-ARM REAR FLY LATERAL RAISE

To start: Standing, hold one side of the band in the left hand with wrist, elbow, and shoulder aligned, and anchor the other end under your left foot.

Instructions:

1. Keep the right hand in place as you raise the left arm to shoulder level, leading with the elbow and squeezing the back and shoulder. Adjust band placement under your foot to increase or decrease tension.

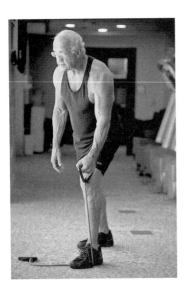 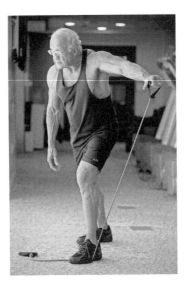

RESISTANCE BAND OVERHEAD PRESS

To start: Stand on the band, holding handles in both hands.

Instructions:

1. Bend arms in "goalpost" position, wrists straight and abs in.

2. Contract the shoulders and straighten arms upward, then lower back down.

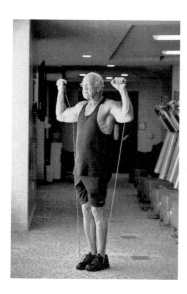 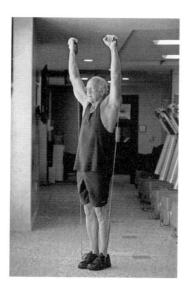

RESISTANCE BAND SQUATS

To start: Stand on the band with feet shoulder width apart, keeping tension on the band by holding a half-bicep curl.

Instructions:

1. Lower into a squat, keeping knees behind toes, and pulling on the band to add tension. Return to start and repeat.

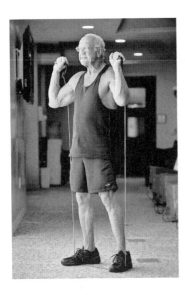 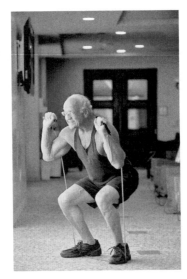

RESISTANCE BAND LUNGES

To start: Stand with right leg forward, left leg back, and band positioned under right leg.

Instructions:

1. Keeping tension on the band by bending elbows, lower into a lunge until both knees are at 90 degrees and your front knee is just behind your toes. Return to start and repeat.

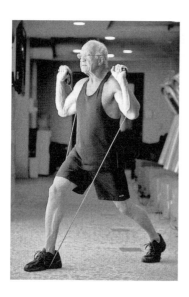 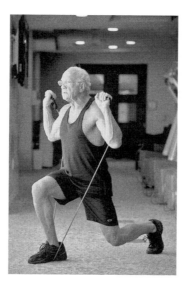

RESISTANCE BAND SIDE STEPS

To start: Stand on the resistance band with your feet at hip distance apart.

Instructions:

1. Take 8 steps to the right, contracting the glutes and outer thigh. Repeat on the other side.

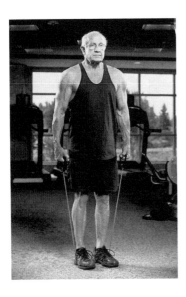 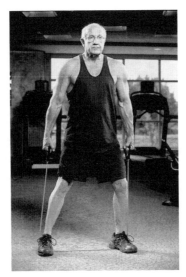

RESISTANCE BAND TRICEPS EXTENSIONS

To start: Hold the band in both hands with your right arm bent so that it's in front of your face and your left arm bent at 90 degrees at your waist.

Instructions:

1. Keeping the right arm locked to hold tension, contract your left triceps to straighten your left arm. Return to start and repeat several times before switching sides.

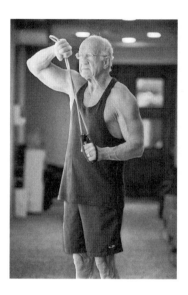 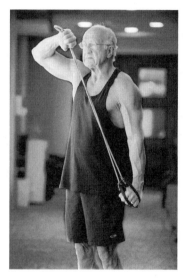

RESISTANCE BAND BICEPS CURLS

To start: Stand on the band and hold handles with palms facing forward.

Instructions:

1. Keeping your abs in and knees slightly bent, bend arms and bring palms toward shoulders in a bicep curl. Position feet wider for more tension. Return to start and repeat.

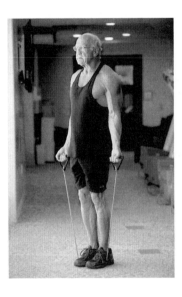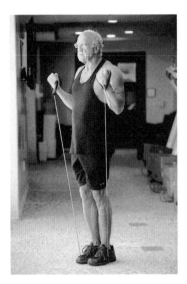

Tips to Make Your Training Perfect

- During the workout you may feel some level of discomfort. If you're in the middle of an exercise and you're feeling a lot of pain, or more pain than you're comfortable with, stop the movement immediately and assess the problem. You should never feel a sharp pain or a sense of searing, burning, or tingling.

- If you have a fever or are feeling nauseated, dizzy, lightheaded, or short of breath you shouldn't be working out. Take the day off. If you're sore from another activity or injury, use caution. My general belief is movement is always better than no movement, but don't push yourself to the point of pain.

- I recommend a light meal before a workout. You don't want to eat anything too heavy before exercising, but you wouldn't want to be empty-bellied either, because you can become dizzy and lightheaded. Sometimes I have a piece of fruit, such as an apple, or a small portion of oatmeal before my session.

- Drink plenty of water throughout your session.

- Communicate with your trainer if you have any kind of restrictions, injuries, or illness so he or she can modify the exercise.

- Choose a trainer who is hands-on—who guides you through each exercise, making sure your form is perfect and assisting you with that last rep if you can't make it on your own.

- Always eat after the workout. You can have a protein shake with half of a banana or an apple. You need to replenish because you do burn more calories than you would expect and you need to provide vital nutrients to your muscles.

- Even if you're not sweating a lot, drink plenty of water during and certainly afterward.

- Wear comfortable clothing that is not too loose. You might want to wear compression shorts underneath regular gym shorts for more support. Keep your shoes and socks on.

- Never hold your breath during weight-lifting. This will inadvertently increase your blood pressure and can cause a stroke. Instead, exhale when you are performing work or producing force against the weight or external resistance. Inhale when reducing force or slowing the weight or external resistance.

- The room you're using should be kept cool.

- You will need a Thera-Band and a clean towel. A Thera-Band is a latex exercise band that is available at most sports equipment stores, your local gym, or on the Internet. They come in eight color-coded levels of resistance.

- Invest in a resistance band Power Station. This is a tool that can help you optimize your resistance band workouts by providing a way to securely attach the band to a solid object, such as a door. These are available at most sporting goods stores or on the Internet.

- When it's time to go to the gym, don't allow any thoughts of not going enter your head. Focus on how great your gym experience makes you feel. Even if you are exhausted, go to the gym! I always feel better when I work out. After a while, going to the gym becomes an enjoyable part of your life and you really look forward to it. If you miss your workout, you'll feel miserable.

- Get a motivated training partner. Statistics show that people who exercise with a friend are more successful at staying with their program. It's especially critical for resistance training: Your partner can spot you on heavier weights and last reps and make sure that you are working out safely. Knowing that someone is waiting for you at the gym can be great motivation to show up and get it done!

FEEDBACK FROM MY FANS

NAME: Bob S.

MESSAGE: Saw you on *The Doctors'* show. Great publicity for you and your dynamite book. I am on my second reading of your best-selling book. You are a great inspiration to me and for every person who reads it. I'm at the gym first thing in the morning, five days a week. I am pushing 77 and feel like a young 30-year-old. I have more muscle today than when I was a 20-year-old playing varsity football at Northern Illinois University. At my age I am still putting on muscle in this old man's body. Thanks to you and continue to inspire us oldies.

. . .

A resistance-training workout takes time to master. Don't rush through the workout, or hurry to move up to heavier weights. It took me 19 weeks of single-minded, grueling exercise to make my initial transformation in 1998. What's more, I train between five and seven days a week to keep my body at this level. I'm telling you this so that you understand that you won't see results overnight, or even in a couple of weeks. However, I know that if you keep at it, you can have the body you've always dreamed of achieving. The sooner you start, the sooner you'll see the results. And when you do, you'll kick yourself for waiting this long!

In the next chapter we'll finish off the workout with my cardio program, in which you'll learn how to burn calories and improve heart function so that you can feel younger longer.

CHAPTER 7

The Life Plan Cardio Workout

Aerobic exercise is all about oxygen. Any activity that increases the heart rate and uses oxygen while using large muscle groups, can be maintained for a prolonged period of time, and is rhythmic in nature is considered an aerobic exercise. Kenneth Cooper, M.D., first popularized the term *aerobic exercise* back in the 1960s, and since then it's been a staple in any good workout program.

Aerobic exercise is also referred to as cardiovascular or "cardio" work because it challenges the cardiovascular system and increases its capacity by overloading the heart and lungs, forcing them to work harder than they do at rest. Your heart's ability to deliver blood (and therefore oxygen) to your working muscles, and your muscles' ability to synthesize large amounts of ATP, enable you to increase your cardiorespiratory fitness. The whole point of aerobics is to improve your ability to consume, transport, and use oxygen in all the thousands of biochemical reactions that go on continuously in your body; reactions that sustain health, prevent disease, and keep you from getting old. Before you start any cardio program you need to be medically cleared to participate. This should include a physical exam and stress test to make sure you have a healthy heart that can safely handle the exercise.

The most important thing to remember about aerobic or cardio exercise is that it is *the only way* to get rid of and keep off the body fat. You can diet from today until the end of time, but if you don't get your heart pumping and your metabolism burning, you are not going to

CARDIO IS WHAT KEEPS ME MOTIVATED

I know that when people see my body, they think I'm a weight-training junkie. But the truth is that it's my cardio workout that keeps me on track. When I slack off on my aerobics, I find that I lose control over my eating, even if I continue with my resistance-training workout. I'm sure this is because my endorphins tank without cardio. Endorphins are produced in the brain during cardio exercise, as well as times when we are excited, in pain, after eating certain foods (like chocolates), and during orgasm. They provide that "runner's high" and overall good feeling, as well as additional energy. So it's the cardio that lifts my mood and keeps me feeling young and healthy, which motivates me to stay with the program.

be able to achieve and maintain fat loss. Stretching/ Pilates will help tone your body and resistance training will bulk you up. But nothing beats aerobic exercise for shedding pounds of fat now and keeping them off for good. The catch is that you have to keep at it.

Aerobic Exercise Protects the Heart

Twenty years ago, researchers and doctors believed that men with heart disease should rest and not overexert themselves in order to stay alive. Now cardiologists are instructing men with heart disease to engage in supervised moderate to vigorous exercise. That's true for both the prevention and treatment of heart disease.

Aerobic exercise is important after a heart attack, angioplasty, bypass surgery, and heart implantation. We now know that regular aerobic exercise prevents age-related loss of endothelial function, the vitally important lining of your heart and blood vessels. What's more, studies show that exercise can restore damaged endothelium to healthy levels in previously sedentary middle-aged and older healthy men. Consistent aerobic exercise also protects the myocardium (your heart muscle). Joseph W. Starnes, Ph.D., head of the Department of Kinesiology at the University of North Carolina in Greensboro, who is internationally known for his cardiovascular research, focuses on the ability of exercise to help protect the heart during a heart attack as well as the effects of exercise, aging, and nutrition on the heart. Before his groundbreaking research, doctors believed that it took weeks or months of regular exercise to gain any degree of protection for the heart. Yet Starnes showed that even a single exercise session stimulates the heart to increase its synthesis of protective proteins, called stress proteins. Within twenty-four hours after exercising, Starnes says, these proteins increase enough to protect the heart against a variety of physical stresses.

Even if you have been diagnosed with heart disease, you must reach a certain threshold of intensity before further cardiac protection is realized. Starnes claims that moderate exercise for 60 minutes can increase your protection greatly. In fact, he thinks exercise intensity above moderate improves the protection gain by only a modest amount.

Regular exercise training protects the heart from injury during a heart attack. However, Starnes's research also shows that exercise-induced cardiac protection is lost once regular exercise is stopped. Approximately a week after you've stopped exercising, you will be back to whatever your pre-exercise level was. So no matter how long or how intensely you've been training, stop and in less than seven days, you're almost back to where you started, and once again you've put your heart back at risk.

This is why it is so important to realize that there are a wide variety of activities that are considered positive, aerobic workouts. Even when you tire of one, don't waste too much time before you choose another. And whatever you choose, make sure that you are moving every single day.

Aerobics Improves the Rest of Your Body

Improves your ability to burn body fat: It is virtually impossible to reduce body fat without cardio exercise. While diet, resistance training, and correcting your hormone deficiencies will help get rid of some body fat, in order to really tap into your fat stores, you must do cardio, and continue doing it for prolonged periods.

Improves your ability to burn calories: Cardio workouts at the proper intensity increase the amount of calories your body needs to carry out its normal functions throughout the day and night, long after you have completed the exercise. This is called your *resting metabolic rate.* The higher the metabolic rate, the more calories you burn every day.

Improves overall energy levels: An increased resting metabolic rate increases your energy, so you are less fatigued during the day and sleep better at night.

Improves sexual function: The more aerobically fit you are, the better your performance is in bed. Working out at an intensity level of 65 to 85 percent maximum heart rate can reverse ED, per a nine-year study published in the August 2000 issue of

Urology by Dr. Irwin Goldstein, Boston University School of Medicine. Investigators found that men who continued or started working out as late as middle age were still able to lower their impotence risk.

Improves nerve transmission: Aerobic exercise improves the interactions of your nervous system with your muscular system, which results in greater strength, coordination, and speed.

Improves the way you look and feel: A recent study published in the January 2010 issue of *Journal of Aging and Physical Activity* showed that consistent aerobic training had a positive effect on muscle mass, power, and strength, which could keep people active and independent for up to two decades longer than with a sedentary lifestyle.

COMBINING AEROBIC EXERCISE WITH THE LIFE PLAN WORKOUT

I believe that a mix of aerobic conditioning, stretching, and strength training is the best exercise program for aging adults. In Chapter 8, you'll see how all three programs come together. I believe the ratio between cardio and resistance training should be about 50/50 for just about any man who wants to achieve and maintain great health, strength, and endurance.

Your Heart Rate Estimates Your Aerobic Potential

Your heart rate (or pulse rate) provides the most valuable information about your level of fitness and your response to exercise. You can use your heart rate to make sure you are training at a level of intensity that will allow you to achieve improved cardiopulmonary health, aerobic conditioning, and fat loss.

The term Heart Rate Max (HR_{max}) is used to define the highest heart rate you can safely achieve. The most accurate way of determining your individual maximum heart rate and how it relates to your oxygen consumption is to have a cardiac stress test monitored by a cardiologist or exercise physiologist. Many doctors, including myself, can perform this test in their offices. Make sure you have this during your evaluation before you start the Life Plan Workout.

There are also various formulas based on your age that can be used to estimate your individual maximum heart rate. These formulations are all significantly less accurate than proper testing. The generally accepted error in age-predicted formulas is plus or minus 10 to 15 beats per minute, and this is due to different inherited characteristics and levels of fitness. However, if you want to get a glimpse of your current health status before you go to see your doctor, you can use the following formula:

$$HR_{max} = 220 - \text{your age}$$

Training Ranges: Heart Rate Zones

Heart rate zone training is the best approach to achieving aerobic fitness. It works for a 74-year-old athlete like me, a 60-year-old with a family history of heart problems, a 45-year-old wanting to improve strength, a 20-year-old who wants to drop body fat and become fit, a 30-year-old who has become sedentary from too much time in front of his computer, and a 50-year-old who is preparing for his second wedding (and honeymoon) and wants to be at his best.

Recent research has shown powerful benefits from exercising your heart in different zones, or rates of exercise, to get maximum benefit. The heart is a muscle that you can strengthen, just like any other muscle. And just like any other, it's a use-it-or-lose-it muscle: If you don't do cardiovascular exercise, your heart will lose its functional ability.

Heart rate zones are expressed as a percentage of your HR_{max} and reflect exercise intensity and the corresponding benefit to your heart. Once you have established your HR_{max} you can calculate your exercise HR for each zone that I have listed below. Your target heart rate (THR) is the desired range of heart rates you need to reach during aerobic training to enable your heart and lungs to get the most benefit from your workout.

Keep in mind, your aerobic capacity—which you can think of as your endurance level—improves much faster if you train closer to 70 to 80 percent rather than 60 percent of your HR_{max} but most men won't be able to start training at this level, especially if they haven't exercised in a while. You may even need to start at 40 percent or 50 percent, depending on your level of fitness, overall health, and current body weight. But don't sweat it: The level that you start with isn't all that relevant. What really matters is that you get started and stick with it. Over time, as your endurance improves, you can gradually increase the intensity. Your body accommodates to both low- and high-intensity workouts by increasing the activity of respiratory enzymes and biochemical reactions in your muscles. Before you know it, you will be able to train at the high end of your target heart rate training zone and look forward to every one of your workouts.

The following list describes typical target heart rate zones. These will help you create an effective workout and gauge the quality of your exercise.

Warmup or healthy heart zone: 50 to 60 percent of your max heart rate. This is a good beginner target zone for someone who is out of shape or has heart problems.

Fitness zone: 60 to 70 percent. This zone will burn more total calories than the warmup zone. Of the calories that are burned, 85 percent will come from existing body fat.

Aerobic zone: 70 to 80 percent. This zone will strengthen your heart and is good for those who want to train for competing in an endurance activity, such as a marathon or triathlon.

Anaerobic zone: 80 to 90 percent. This zone will improve your cardiorespiratory system and will increase your ability to fight fatigue. This zone burns only about 15 percent of its calories from fat during the exercise session, but fat calories continue to be burned for several hours after the session. The goal is to train at this level for 15 to 25 minutes during each workout to get maximum cardiovascular benefit.

Max effort zone: 90 to 100 percent. This zone will burn the highest number of calories and is very intense. Most men can stay in this zone for only a few seconds to a minute or two at most. There is a high risk for injury when training at this zone, and it is not part of the basic Life Plan workouts. To train at this zone, you'll need to master the highest-level workout in my first book, *The Life Plan.*

Target Heart Rate Training Zone

Ideally, you should wear a heart rate monitor during the cardio portion of your exercise, to ensure that you are at an efficient and safe heart rate zone. The newest pieces of exercise equipment, from treadmills to elliptical trainers to stationary bicycles, include a way to detect this information. Or, you can calculate your target heart rate (THR) with the Karvonen Method equation. To determine your resting heart rate (HR_{rest}), take your pulse when you are at rest: awake but lying down. The best way to do this is to check it three mornings in a row just after waking up. Add all of them together and divide by three to get your average HR_{rest}. The lower your resting heart rate, the more fit you are. Typical resting heart rates in men are in the 60 to 80 beats per minute (bpm) range. Conditioned athletes have resting heart rates below 60 bpm. My resting heart rate is typically in the mid to upper 50s. Here is an example that will help you calculate your target heart rate training zone based on your resting heart rate.

$$THR = (HR_{max} - HR_{rest}) \times (\text{Training Range \%}) + HR_{rest}$$

For example, here are my numbers:

Target Heart Rate = 60% intensity: $(146-55) \times (0.60) + 55 = 109$ bpm

Target Heart Rate = 85% intensity: $(146-55) \times (0.85) + 55 = 132$ bpm

Each time I train I need to make sure that my heart rate is somewhere between 125 bpm and 135 bpm to be in a training zone that will enable my heart and lungs to receive the most benefit.

PAY ATTENTION TO YOUR HEART RATE RECOVERY

Your heart rate should recover quickly to your pre-exercise level within two minutes following your workout. A healthy heart rate recovery is a decrease in your pulse of 50 to 65 beats per minute at two minutes after you exercise. An abnormal heart rate recovery is a failure to decrease your heart rate by more than 20 beats per minute two minutes after you exercise. If your recovery heart rate falls into the abnormal category, it could simply mean that you are out of shape and deconditioned, or it could be a sign of a more serious heart condition. While a general recovery heart rate test can be done on your own or in a gym, you should have a formal stress test administered by a cardiologist if you are over 45, have a family history of heart disease, experience shortness of breath, chest pain, discomfort or dizziness during exercise, or have an abnormal heart rate recovery like that I described above.

You Need to Burn 1,000 to 2,000 Calories per Week

The last piece of the cardio workout puzzle is: Just how much cardio exercise do we need? I recommend that men need to burn 1,000 to 2,000 calories (kilocalories) per week doing cardio. Again, the newest cardio equipment at your local gym can calculate this right on the machine. But if you want to be a runner or a swimmer, you'll need to calculate this yourself in order to figure out just how long your cardio sessions need to be each week to effectively condition your heart and lungs and achieve a lean, fit, sexy body.

In order to do this, you'll need access to a calorie calculator, on which you can determine your caloric expenditure during exercise. These offer a very rough estimate, but are a good way to get basic information. They allow you to plug in your weight and either the distance you plan on traveling or the minutes you will be doing a particular exercise. From there, you can increase your expenditure by increasing either of these variables. My trainer, Rod Stanley, features the distance model on his website, www.rpmfit.com/_Calories_Burned_Calculator_.html, or go with a time-oriented model at www.healthstatus.com/calculate/cbc.

High-Intensity Interval Training

Interval training or high-intensity interval training (HIIT) is an exercise strategy that is very attractive to busy men because it improves performance with short training sessions lasting from 4 to 35 minutes. HIIT is defined as high-intensity work alternated with rest or periods of low-intensity work. These bursts of high-intensity training are at the anaerobic zone (80 to 90 percent of max heart rate). During the periods of low intensity, your heart rate comes back down to around 50 percent of your max heart rate. This training involves major muscle groups such as your legs, back, and arms for people who are serious about dropping body fat and improving the functional capacity of their cardiovascular and pulmonary systems. HIIT sessions lasting 20 to 25 minutes with a 5-minute warmup and a 5-minute cooldown period are the best way to achieve heart and lung protection and burn body fat. This is what I have been doing for the past three years, and I can assure you it works.

HIIT is very physically demanding and isn't for everybody. If you have existing cardiovascular issues or other health concerns that limit your ability to exercise intensely, or if you are new to aerobic training, HIIT may not be right for you now, but you will be able to work up to it. It is not advised for the deconditioned until a stress test has been performed and you have been medically cleared for high-intensity cardio training.

Interval training can be performed with any modality of cardio exercise and is very simple to do. For example, if you are on a treadmill or exercise bicycle, just start out at a low level and once you are warmed up (3–5 minutes), advance the level of difficulty by adding 1 or 2 minutes of higher-intensity intervals interspersed with low-level rest periods of 1 minute. Just keep increasing your high-intensity level of work until you get to the percentage of your target heart rate you want to work at (80 to 90 percent) and stay there. (For 1 to 2 minutes or as long as you can maintain this intensity. If you are able to hold the top intensity for a period longer than 2 minutes, then you are not training hard enough and should raise your heart rate a few beats per minute.) When you have performed 2 to 6 of these intervals, it's time for a 5-minute cooldown. You will need a heart rate monitor to gauge the intensity of your workouts.

Most high-intensity interval workouts take around 20 to 35 minutes, including warmup and cooldown. If you like to listen to music while you exercise, you can set up musical cues to prompt you when to speed up or slow down. You can actually download fast songs separated by slower songs to create the perfect HIIT playlist. As your level of fitness improves, you can reprogram your music appropriately.

The Components of a Good Cardio Program

I use the acronym FITT to outline all of the areas you need to consider for your program.

F—**Frequency:** How many days will you need to do cardio work in order to burn 1,000 to 2,000 calories? I suggest that you start with a 3-day program, working up to a 5-day program. You may be able to burn only 1,000 calories a week when you start, but don't be discouraged: If you keep at it, you'll quickly be able to add time and burn more body fat.

I—**Intensity:** Train at a heart rate that is appropriate for your goals. Start easy and increase your level of intensity. Remember, this is not a 12-week program, it is a lifetime program. "Train Safely" is the Life Plan motto.

T—**Time:** How much time will you need to spend during each cardio session? Again, this can increase as you become more aerobically fit.

T—Type: Aerobic exercise has almost an unlimited number of forms, including running, swimming, racquetball, tennis, bicycling, rowing, calisthenics, martial arts, stair climbing, jumping rope, cross-country skiing, fencing; the list goes on and on and includes any activity that increases heart rate and oxygen uptake for a prolonged time period. Find at least two or three cardio activities you already enjoy that can be switched around depending on your time and availability of training partners and facilities (courts, pools, gyms, and so on). In *The Life Plan*, I use a modified version of the Metabolic Equivalents, or METs, table, to list dozens of activities that are considered cardiovascular workouts. This table compares the activities so that you can see which ones offer the biggest bang for the buck. But you can guess that tennis expends more energy than bowling, or that running or swimming is more active than a stroll on the beach.

Your beginning cardio program may look something like this:

Frequency	Intensity	Time	Type
3 days a week	60%–70% of your HR_{max}	30 minutes	cycling

After two weeks, revisit the FITT principle and increase your cardio program. A method that I commonly use is:

Week 3: Increase **Frequency**

Week 4: Increase **Intensity**

Week 5: Increase **Time**

Week 6: Change **Type**

Be sure to keep accurate records of your HR_{max} and heart rate recovery in the journal in Chapter 8. You will know when you are ready to move into the next phase of your training when your workouts become too easy, your HR_{max} is lower, or your heart rate recovery becomes faster. If you move ahead and find that you are not ready, don't get discouraged. Just go back to where you were, and in a week or so you will be able to comfortably move to the next level. Don't forget, this is not a 12-week program, this program is a Life Plan: You don't have to rush to the next level until you are completely ready.

Mastering a Cardio Workout

I perform 40 to 50 minutes of cardio five times a week, either swimming or on an exercise bike. When I bike, I either join a spin class or work out alone at my home on my stationary bike. I enjoy these activities because I can program or follow along with a high-intensity interval training session. I have been doing this for several years and find it is the best way to achieve heart and lung protection and burn body fat. They are also very safe choices because it's difficult (but not impossible) to fall off a stationary bike.

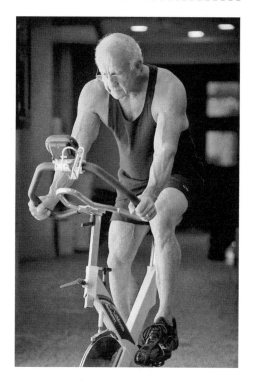

Spin classes have been a joy for me because I like the social aspect of it, and believe it or not, I enjoy the music. They are typically held in a separate spin studio within a gym, or in a freestanding location. The class features stationary bikes in a room with a trainer, who choreographs the class along with music to keep everyone motivated. Some classes feature video that's synced in as well.

One of the great things about spinning is that it is adaptable to any fitness level: It's not a competition. You can go at your own pace by controlling the resistance on your bike. If you're a first-timer, let the instructor know so that he or she can make sure your bike is properly adjusted. Your seat should be high enough that your knees are only slightly bent.

When I can't make a spin class, I work out on a stationary bicycle (a LifeCycle, if you can believe it!) or swim. I find that the time goes by quickly, and the workouts are as intense as I want them to be. I follow an interval-training program that I can modify in the pool or on the bike as I go. The LifeCycle, the first computerized indoor cycle, was developed in the mid-1960s. Your local gym may have two varieties: the upright and recumbent, or leaning back, positions. Most stationary bikes have electronically controlled resistance, heart rate and caloric output monitors, entertainment consoles, computerized workout programs, and even virtual reality workouts that can simulate cycling up and down hills and on flat terrain.

Tips to Make Spinning, Cycling, or Swimming a Success

- During the workout you may feel some level of discomfort in your legs or arms, or if you overexert and cannot catch your breath. If you're in the middle of group exercise and you're feeling a lot of pain, stop immediately and assess the problem.

- If you have a fever or are feeling nauseated, dizzy, lightheaded, or short of breath you shouldn't be working out. Take the day off.

- If you're sore from another activity or injury, use caution. My general belief is movement is always better than no movement, but don't push yourself to the point of pain.

- I recommend a light meal before a workout. You don't want to eat anything too heavy before exercising, but you wouldn't want to be empty-bellied either, because you can become dizzy and lightheaded. Sometimes I have a piece of fruit, such as an apple, or a small portion of oatmeal before my practice.

- Communicate with your class leader if you have any kind of restrictions, injuries, or illness so he or she can modify the bike for you.

- Always eat after the workout. You can have a protein shake or an apple, depending on how you feel. The typical caloric deficit in a one-hour session is roughly 400–600 calories.

- You'll be sweating a lot, especially if you are a beginner. That's why it's important to drink lots of water during and certainly afterward.

- Comfortable workout attire is all you need to get started for most cardio programs. Padded cycling shorts and moisture-wicking tops will make your workout more comfortable if you are going to follow the spinning/cycling program.

- Most aerobic activity requires shoes and socks (except for swimming), and often requires special shoes that help you perform better. For example, cycling shoes are made with very stiff soles that enable more powerful pedal strokes. Speak with an instructor to help you pick out the right shoes for your chosen activity.

- Watch out for numbness in the feet during exercise. This is most likely caused by restricted blood flow due to shoes, shoelaces, or toe straps that are too tight. Loosening laces and straps often solves the problem. If this doesn't help, consider foam insoles or front-ended orthotics. They can provide relief by redistributing pressure toward the balls of your feet.

- A heart rate monitor will help you get the most from every workout. This is an easy and inexpensive purchase that can be made online or in any quality sporting goods store. Look for one with a waist belt component.

- During your cardio workouts it's important to continue to remain relaxed. You can accomplish this by breathing deeply and slowly and avoiding shallow breaths. Concentrate on your breathing and keep it well controlled. Breathe in through the nose and out through the mouth.

- Keep your neck and shoulders relaxed. It's easy to tense up when you are doing cardio, and the next thing you know your shoulders will be riding up near your ears. Practice keeping them down and you'll be more comfortable during and after your workout.

- The room you're using should be kept cool.

- If you are a beginner, have the instructor coach you on the proper adjustment for the bike to ensure the most comfortable ride possible. Proper bike adjustment will also help you perform better by eliminating unnecessary performance-hindering movements throughout the class. Remember, everyone in the class has been a beginner at some point: Don't be afraid to ask for help.

- Exercise to music whenever possible, and pick a tempo that motivates you.

- When I work out at home on my LifeCycle I use ear buds and catch up on action TV series (or old favorites), such as *24, Prison Break, The Shield, The Wire, The Unit*, or *Sons of Anarchy*. The pace of these programs really motivates my performance.

The Life Plan Gym Cardio Spinning/Cycling Workout

If you are taking a spin class, show this workout to your instructor and see if he or she can work with the program, or suggest a specific class or time that most closely matches the workout. If you are using a stationary bike outside of a class, ask a trainer to help you set up the bike's computer programming to mimic these suggestions.

This workout begins with Phase 1, a 20-minute program, including your warmup and cooldown. Begin by completing the first workout 3 times a week. Then, add days until you get to a routine where you are doing cardio 5 days a week. At that point you can start adding minutes, moving to Phase 2, which adds just 6 minutes to the workout. Phase 3 is the final phase that includes another 5 minutes. At that point you will be doing cardio for 30 minutes, 5 days a week.

This program is based on an intensity scale that is rated from 1 to 10, in which 1 equals very easy and 10 equals very hard (barely doable). You can fairly easily transfer these levels to the intensity levels on the exercise equipment. So if there are 25 levels on the bike and your level of perceived exertion is about 7, then you can start at Level 13 and work your way up.

Phase 1: Beginners

Warmup Start at Level 2 or 3, which should be **40–50%** THR, and then gradually increase your level of intensity over a 3- to 5-minute period until you reach moderate intensity, where you'll begin your workout.

- Level 4: moderate resistance, stay seated. You should at least be **50–60%** THR.

- 1 minute at 100 RPMs

- 1 minute at 110 RPMs

- 1 minute all-out effort

- Level 5: remain seated. You should at least be **60–70%** THR.

- 1 minute at 100 RPMs

- 1 minute at 110 RPMs

- 1 minute all-out effort

- **1 minute seated recovery Level 2**

- Level 5: seated. You will approach **70–80%** THR.

- 1 minute at 100 RPMs

- 1 minute at 110 RPMs

- 1 minute all-out effort

- Level 6: standing. You will approach **80%-plus** THR.

- 1 minute at 80–90 RPMs

- 1 minute at 90–100 RPMs

- 1 minute all-out effort

- **1 minute seated recovery Level 2**

Beginners stop here and go into a 3-minute recovery/cooldown. Reduce your effort to achieve 40% THR until your heart rate has returned to resting levels. Your goal should be to drop to Level 4 and then gradually decrease to Level 1 for the last minute of your cooldown.

- 6 minutes cardio static stretching after cooldown

Phase 2: Intermediate/Advanced Riders Continue

- Level 6: seated. You should approach **80–90%** THR.

- 1 minute at 80–90 RPMs

- 1 minute at 90–100 RPMs

- 1 minute all-out effort

- Level 7: standing. You should maintain **80–90%** THR.

- 1 minute at 80–90 RPMs

- 1 minute at 90–100 RPMs

- 1 minute all-out effort

Intermediate riders stop here and go into a 3-minute recovery/cooldown. Reduce your effort to achieve 40% THR until heart rate has returned to resting levels. Your goal should be to drop to Level 4 and then gradually decrease to Level 1 for the last minute of your cooldown.

- 6 minutes cardio static stretching after cooldown

Phase 3: Advanced Riders Continue

- **1 minute recovery seated Level 2**

- Level 7: seated. You should be at least **80–90%** THR.

- 1 minute at 80–90 RPMs

- 1 minute standing all-out effort

- Level 8: standing. Aim for **90–100%** THR.

- 1 minute at 80–90 RPMs

- 1 minute standing all-out effort

- 3-minute recovery/cooldown. Reduce your effort to achieve 40% THR until heart rate has returned to resting levels. Your goal should be to drop to Level 4 and then gradually decrease to Level 1 for the last minute of your cooldown.

- 6 minutes cardio static stretching after cooldown

The At-Home Cardio Workout

You can do the following workout in your home. If you have any home gym equipment, such as a stationary bicycle or treadmill, you can use the workout above: It will work with almost any type of cardio equipment, including elliptical trainers and rowing machines.

Another option is to create a route in your neighborhood where you can replicate a 20-minute walk, and follow the directions below to pick up speed or slow down as necessary. As you become fit and your endurance increases, add 5-minute increments to the workout, evenly spacing the time between intervals. Continue adding minutes until you get up to a 40-minute workout, 3 times a week. Then, add days until you get to a routine in which you are doing cardio 5 days a week.

Interval Training in the Pool

It's easy to create an interval training session in a pool environment. All you need is access to a pace clock, or a water proof wrist watch with a second hand. I do 50-meter intervals and rest for 10 to 20 seconds between each one. Then I do two or three 100s with a rest period of 30 to 45 seconds between each one. If I am really feeling good, I will then do one or two 200s with a rest period of 60 to 90 seconds between each one. Then I end up with a slow 100 yards to cool down.

Interval Training at Home

Begin with 20 minutes, 3 times a week.

- 5 minutes warmup. This a fairly easy pace starting at low intensity and keeping your heart rate at about 40–50 percent of your THR. You will mentally and physically prepare your body to work by gradually increasing your pace to moderate intensity (60–70 percent THR). Your heart rate should begin to increase during the 4th and 5th minutes. Then advance into the following.

- 30 seconds moderate intensity (60–70 percent THR), 1 minute low intensity (40–50 percent THR).

- 45 seconds moderate intensity (60–70 percent THR), 1 minute low intensity (40–50 percent THR).

- 60 seconds moderate intensity (60–70 percent THR), 1 minute low intensity (40–50 percent THR).

- 60 seconds moderate intensity (60–70 percent THR), 1 minute low intensity (40–50 percent THR).

- 90 seconds moderate intensity (60–70 percent THR), 1 minute low intensity (40–50 percent THR).

- 90 seconds moderate intensity (60–70 percent THR), 1 minute low intensity (40–50 percent THR).

- 90 seconds moderate intensity (60–70 percent THR), 1 minute low intensity (40–50 percent THR).

- 90 seconds moderate intensity (60–70 percent THR), 1 minute low intensity (40–50 percent THR).

- 60 seconds high intensity (70–80 percent THR), 1 minute low intensity (40–50 percent THR).

- 60 seconds high intensity (70–80 percent THR), 1 minute low intensity (40–50 percent THR).

- 45 seconds high intensity (70–80 percent THR), 1 minute low intensity (40–50 percent THR).

- 30 seconds high intensity (70–80 percent THR), 30 seconds low intensity (40–50 percent THR).

- 5 minutes cooldown. Reduce your effort to achieve 40 percent THR until heart rate has returned to resting levels.

- 6 minutes static stretching after cooldown (see below).

The Post-Cardio Static Stretch Routine

After any type of cardio workout, take a few minutes for some static stretching. This is very similar to the Pilates stretching, but these particular exercises are meant to loosen the areas of the body that become tight during a typical cardio workout, particularly the legs. Each of the following static stretch positions should be held for 20 to 30 seconds and repeated three to five times with a complete relaxation of the muscle between each repetition. The stretches should be done in a gentle and relaxed motion, moving just to the point where you can feel a stretch in the muscles you are working, and not in the other muscles that you are not working. For example, if you are stretching your calves, you should not feel a pull in your back.

NECK STRETCH

To start: Begin by standing with feet shoulder width apart.

Instructions:

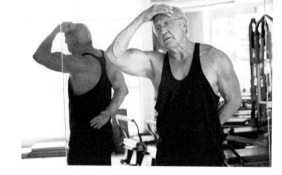

1. Take right hand and place it on left side of your forehead just above the eyebrow.

2. Place the left arm behind your back with your hand in the middle of your back while rolling your left shoulder back.

3. Applying slight pressure, turn your head to the right until you feel a stretch on the left side of the neck.

4. Hold for 20–30 seconds, then rest and repeat on the other side.

UPPER BACK STRETCH

To start: Start with your right hand extended forward and grasp a piece of exercise equipment. Stand with feet shoulder width apart, knees slightly bent and toes pointed forward.

Instructions:

1. Lean your body backward and stretch your right upper back and lat.

2. Hold this stretch for 20–30 seconds, then relax.

3. Repeat on the other side.

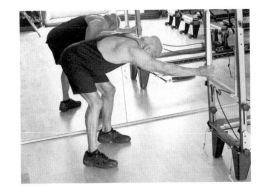

SHOULDER STRETCH

To start: Stand with feet shoulder width apart, knees slightly bent and toes pointed forward.

Instructions:

1. Place your left arm across your body at shoulder height and gently pull it toward your right shoulder with your right hand.

2. Continue holding your left arm either above or below the elbow.

3. Look over your left shoulder to deepen the stretch.

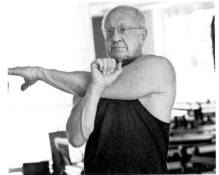

4. Hold for 20–30 seconds, then rest and repeat on the other side.

THORACIC SPINE STRETCH

To start: Kneel on the floor on all fours with your knees under your hips and hands under your shoulders.

Instructions:

1. Keeping palms flat on the floor, contract the abs to bring head, neck, and back into alignment.

2. Tilt the hip bones toward the ceiling while drawing shoulders back and down.

3. Tuck the chin and round your back until you feel a stretch down your spine.

4. Hold for 20–30 seconds, then relax and repeat.

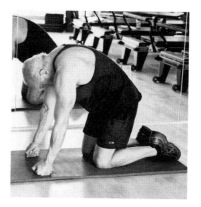

LOWER BACK STRETCH

To start: Lie on your back with your knees bent and feet flat on the floor.

Instructions:

1. Place both hands on top of your right and left shin, just below the knee, and gently pull your knees up into your chest.

2. For a deeper stretch, straighten your left leg out along the floor.

3. Hold for 20–30 seconds, then rest and repeat on the other side.

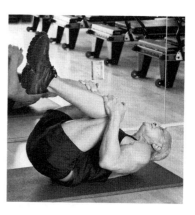

HIP FLEXOR STRETCH

To start: Stand with your right leg forward and left leg back.

Instructions:

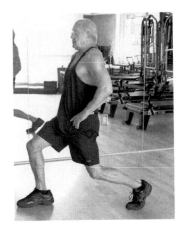

1. Keep your torso erect and slightly point your left foot toward your right foot.

2. Keep your left foot on the floor. Push the hips forward, allowing your right knee to bend.

3. Hold for 20–30 seconds and repeat on the other side.

QUAD STRETCH

To start: Lie on a mat facedown and place your left hand between your forehead and the floor.

Instructions:

1. Keeping hips on the floor, bring your right leg up behind you and grab your foot.

2. Keep your head down and neck relaxed.

3. Hold for 20–30 seconds and repeat with the left leg.

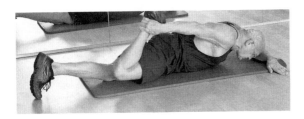

OUTER THIGH STRETCH

To start: Sit on the floor with your left leg straight out in front of you and right leg bent.

Instructions:

1. Cross the bent right leg over the left and place your right foot flat on the floor.

2. Keeping your back straight, grasp your outer right thigh, pulling it to the left while slowly twisting your upper body to the right as you look over your right shoulder.

3. Hold for 20–30 seconds, then rest and repeat on the other side.

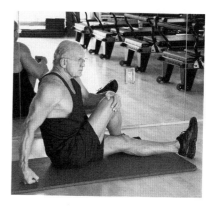

ADDUCTOR STRETCH

To start: Stand with legs slightly wider than shoulder width apart, feet pointed straight ahead.

Instructions:

1. Shift your weight onto your left leg while bending your knee, keeping your right leg extended.

2. Rotate upper body in direction of your left leg until the stretch is felt in the inner thigh of the right leg.

3. Hold for 20–30 seconds, then rest and repeat on the other side.

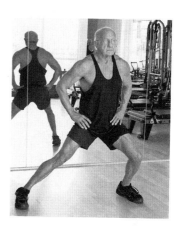

CALF STRETCH

To start: Stand with your right leg behind you, keeping both feet flat on the floor and your right knee straight.

Instructions:

1. Lean slightly forward until you feel tension in the calf of the extended leg. You may also place your hands on a wall or table for support.

2. Hold for 20–30 seconds and repeat on the other side.

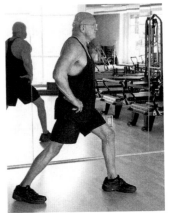

MEET DAVE

I'm 53 years old, five foot nine. My weight has fluctuated between 235 and 245 pounds, and I'm diabetic, taking prescription medication every day. I had been warned that my triglycerides were high, but when I came in to meet Dr. Life for the first time my chief complaint was that I was really tired all the time. Well, I got my blood tests back and my triglycerides were over 1,100, and I actually broke out into a sweat: I had been watching my diet for the past six months and thought I was doing well. But Dr. Life very calmly said, "Dave, you're very fortunate that you came in when you did." I knew right then that the other part of that sentence that he didn't say out loud was "Dave, you could be dead." And that's what motivated me to finally make the commitment to change.

I'm a banker, and you can imagine that the past few years have been really stressful. On a scale between 1 and 10, my stress level was probably about a 7, 8, or 9. I took a nap every day after work, and on the weekends I'd just crash. I'd never have enough energy and on the weekends I'd just try to catch up so that I could have the energy to go back to work the following week. When I was really stressed I would go for comfort foods and sleep, just trying to get through the day and eat and sleep. Exercise was not a part of my life at all.

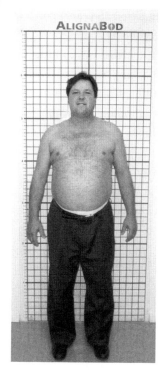

So far, it's been about six weeks that I've been following the Life Plan and I'm already feeling fantastic. I feel like I felt 20 years ago when I was playing basketball and racquetball all the time, and my energy level is back. I've already lost 20 pounds, but what's more important is that I don't have to take naps anymore. I'm working out every day, and my diet has totally changed.

The cardio and the resistance training are so important to me, but the results I'm seeing with the cardio are the most impressive. I've been working out on the treadmill. I set it to where I warm up for 2–3 minutes, then I get to a 9 percent incline and try to keep that at a little more than 3 miles per hour, and if I can do that at the end of about 40 minutes I've burned off about 400 calories, and my heart rate is between 150 and 160. I don't really take any breaks during the workout. I'm just walking up that hill as hard as I can. The first 3 or 4 minutes are pretty easy, and then from about 5 minutes through the next 15 minutes it's really a challenge. But

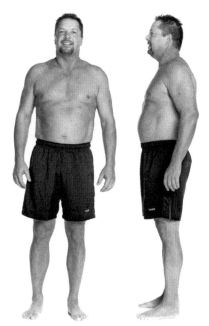

I just keep looking at the calories on the machine that I've burned off and I put my head down and keep going. Then once I get to 15–20 minutes the workout gets pretty easy, and by the time I get to the end I'm worn out. I look at how many calories I've burned and I can finally relax and do my cooldown.

I'm constantly telling myself that there's no way I'm going to fail. All my friends know that I'm doing this. I just keep looking at my "before" pictures and I know I'm just not going back there. They are really quite eye-opening: When I look at them I can hardly believe that is me. There's no way I'm going back to the way I used to be.

I'd like to get below 200 pounds. I weighed 185 when I got married 28 years ago, and I'd like to get back to where I was. I'm surprised that the weight isn't coming off quicker, but at the same time I know that I'm building muscle. The inches are coming off but they're being replaced by more muscle. That's a little frustrating because I think if I was just doing cardio then I would have lost more weight, but I can also see that this program is transforming my body. I've got a friend right now who weighs about the same as me and he does two hours of cardio a day and he's still looks fat and chubby. His body is not toning up the same way mine is.

The best motivation for me is Dr. Life himself. He's living proof that his program works. When I look at him all I think is that I want to be like him in 20 years.

· · ·

Now that you have been introduced to all three components of the Life Plan workout, let's see how you can put them together into a weekly exercise program that you'll love to follow. You'll see in just a week how easy it is to master this. Once you do, you'll leave all your old excuses behind and be excited to wake up each day and get moving.

CHAPTER 8

Mastering the Life Plan Journal

- -

As in everything else in life, success can be found in the details. I'm much better at sticking to a diet and exercise program if I write down every day exactly what I've accomplished. This works for me on several levels. First, it makes me accountable for everything that I put into my mouth, and every minute at the gym. I then have a record to refer to so that I can track my success, and be able to see why some weeks were more effective than others. Second, if I have an illness or injury, I can keep a record to help me better understand what's going on and how my recovery is progressing, and, if necessary, share with my doctor. Third, tracking my progress provides a sense of satisfaction at the end of each day when I recognize that I was able to stay on the right track.

This chapter provides two different journals: one for the diet and one for the exercise program. You can photocopy these pages or download them from my website, www.drlife.com. Put a week's worth of sheets in a binder or fold them in your wallet, and bring them with you wherever you go. You can also keep this information on your smartphone or iPad. I like to fill in the information as I go throughout the day, instead of trying to remember before bedtime what I ate or which exercises I performed. And by recording my meals right after I eat them, I can see if I need to make small adjustments later on in the day. For example, if I had to eat breakfast out of the house, and the omelet I ordered at the restaurant was made with three eggs instead of two, I can choose a lower-calorie snack during the day to compensate.

Setting Goals

It's crucial to stick with this program for at least 12 weeks: four weeks on the Basic Health Diet and then another eight weeks on either the Fat-Burning or Heart Health program. It generally takes that long just for your brain to create new habits and your body to get into the swing of exercise and clean eating. By then you will see significant changes to your physique. After the first six weeks you'll be able to evaluate your progress and then determine if you want to keep going on this program or move to a higher level in this book, or switch to the one outlined in *The Life Plan*.

Before you begin, it's a good idea to see where you want to go. If you've talked to your doctor, he or she may have a specific weight-loss goal in mind. You might have a photo of when you were looking your best, from a wedding or family affair. Or you might just remember how you used to feel, and want to recapture that state of health.

I find that the best way to achieve goals is to set reasonable expectations. Don't start too high: Setting a goal of losing 30 pounds or more is admirable, but it's going to take time, and you may become frustrated along the way and just plain quit. Instead, let's look short term. By focusing on small, achievable goals you can recalibrate as you go, setting new, attainable objectives every month. For example, a first goal could be losing 10 pounds. Once you've accomplished that, move to a larger weight-loss goal that is still within a reasonable range. A second goal could be to keep those 10 pounds off and lose another 5.

A common system that is used for goal setting is the SMART system.

Specific: Set a specific yet broad, goal such as losing fat, gaining muscle, sports performance, or even just improving your general health.

Measurable: A measurable goal is one for which you can objectively determine your success. A measurable goal would be to perform the Life Plan Cardio Workout at least three times per week, with the goal of adding another day in two weeks. Another measurable goal is to lose five pounds in two weeks.

Achievable: Do you have the mind-set, time, and physical requirements necessary for meeting your goals? Make sure you have everything you'll need to follow the program on hand before you begin. That means doing a full food shop, locating the right clothes for working out, and purchasing any equipment necessary, such as the exercise bands or a heart rate monitor. Check your calendar: Are you able to block out the time necessary to complete the workout every day? Work with your schedule instead of working against it, and make sure to schedule your workout into your daily routine, rather than waiting for free time to just appear.

Reasonable: Remember, you won't look like me after just one week of exercise and dieting, no matter how hard you try. Modify your expectations to look for reasonable results after the first two weeks, and not before.

Timed: Set a date in the future when you would like to achieve your largest goal. It may take you a few months to get there, but that's okay. Set the date in stone and don't change it once you have it set.

Calculating Weight-Loss Goals

Once you have your goal in mind, let's check to see if it's reasonable. First, you need to know your current weight. Simple enough: Step on a reliable scale and record that number right here. This will help you refer back to see exactly how much weight you lost since the beginning of the program. Use a marker or a pen, because you'll want to see this number for a long time. Then, record your current height.

Current weight: _____

Height: _____

You need both of these numbers to determine your body mass index, or BMI, a mathematical formula for determining whether you are overweight. This index is calculated by multiplying your weight by 705, dividing the result by your height in inches, and then dividing again by your height in inches. If your BMI is between 25 and 30 you are considered heavy, and if it is greater than 30 you're obese.

For example, I weigh 188 pounds and I'm 5 feet 10 inches tall (70 inches). My BMI equation is:

$$[(188 \times 705) \div 70] = 27$$

which puts me near the top end of the overweight range—almost obese!

Even though BMI is considered important information, I take it with a grain of salt. First of all, while BMI is a good predictor of health when we are looking at large populations, it doesn't work so well when we are assessing individuals, as you can see from my example. Every man who is muscular is likely to be considered at least overweight according to the BMI, even if he is lean—because of his increased muscle weight. Worse, there are plenty of men who have a great BMI but have way too much fat and very little muscle mass. These guys are now known as having Normal Weight Obese Syndrome—light on muscle and heavy on fat. And as you know, carrying around too much body fat profoundly influences our health, physical and mental performance, and appearance.

So do the math for yourself and record the results, but as you'll learn, there are better ways to determine how fit you really are.

Record your initial BMI below, then recalculate in six weeks:

BMI: _____ Date: _____

BMI six weeks later: _____ Date: _____

Beyond BMI: Percentage Body Fat Measurements

Many doctors agree with me that the measurement we should be focusing on is our percent body fat. This can help us determine our ideal body weight, degree of fatness, and risk for disease. The most accurate way to measure body fat percentage is with a DEXA scan, which many doctors, including myself, can perform right in their office. A DEXA scan tells how many grams of muscle tissue you have, as well as your bone density. It can also track gains in muscle mass resulting from this type of fat-loss/muscle-building program.

In the following table, I have listed the percentages of body fat for men according to their age that correlate with excellent to poor health/fitness ratings. Body fat of more than 25 percent puts men in the obese, high-health-risk category. As a general rule, no man at any age should have greater than 15 percent body fat if he wants to remain optimally fit and healthy. At age 74, I work very hard at keeping my body fat below 10 percent. I also know that when my body fat is this low I feel the best, have far greater energy, move better, think better, look the best, and have the lowest risk for disease.

PERCENTAGE OF BODY FAT FOR MEN

Health/Fitness Rating	Age yrs. 20–29	30–39	40–49	50–59	60+
Excellent	<11	<12	<14	<15	<16
Good	11–13	12–14	14–16	15–17	16–18
Average	14–20	15–21	17–23	18–24	19–25
Fair	21–23	22–24	24–26	25–27	26–28
Poor	>23	>24	>26	>27	>28

It is extremely difficult to measure body fat percentage, and impossible to do it on your own. Many personal trainers, or your doctor, can measure your body fat using a tool called a *skin-fold caliper*. However, the results are only as good as the tester: You must have a second person assist you in measuring the thickness of your skin folds at various sites on your body. The measurements are then plugged into an equation to determine your body fat percentage, and there are more than 100 different calculations to choose from.

However, you can easily work with a trainer or your doctor to measure the most common sites, and then retake these measurements after you've been following the program. This way, you'll be able to track your success without having to deal with the variables that make this testing difficult and inaccurate.

Record skin-fold testing for each of these sites now, and then test again in six weeks. Measure only one side of the body, and be consistent later by remeasuring the same side. Remember that your abdominal area is the first place you gain fat . . . and the last place you drop the fat. But don't get discouraged, because it will ultimately disappear if you are consistent with your workout program and eat clean.

Right tricep: _____ Date: _____

Right bicep: _____ Date: _____

Abdomen: _____ Date: _____

Right thigh: _____ Date: _____

Right calf: _____ Date: _____

Sizing Up Your Spare Tire

A second measurement to record is your waist circumference. This alone has been shown to be a better predictor of future heart attacks and Type 2 diabetes than body mass index. It is very easy to determine if you have too much intra-abdominal fat (fat inside your belly), and you don't need any fancy, high-priced laboratory tests to do it. All you need is an inexpensive cloth tape measure. Simply measure your waist circumference. And I don't mean the "low waist," where most of us wear our pants, but rather the "high waist"—one inch above your belly button, where you are the largest. If your waist circumference is 40 inches or greater your risk for life-threatening disease increases dramatically.

Waist circumference: _____ Date: _____

Six-week measurement: _____ Date: _____

Now fill in the following short- and long-term goals, and the dates you would like to achieve them:

Today's date: _____

Largest goal: _____ Date: _____

Two-week goal: _____ Date: _____

Four-week Goal: _____ Date: _____

Six-week Goal: _____ Date: _____

Take Photos Frequently

During my transformation, my best motivator was the "before" photo that I sent to the Body-*for*-LIFE competition. Every time I didn't feel like dieting or exercising, I would just look at that photo of myself and remember how much I didn't want to be that man anymore.

Take front and side-view photos of yourself as if you were getting ready to go to the beach: no top, just bathing trunks. Keep these photos in your cell phone or in your wallet and look at them often. Every week, take another set wearing the same bathing suit. These photos will become an amazing record of what you will achieve by following this program. Trust me; you will cherish each and every one after you have reached your ultimate goal of a lean, muscular body. I almost threw away my "boat picture" that's featured on the cover of my first book. I'm really glad I didn't!

The Life Plan Food Journal

Record each of your five meals every day on the grid below. You can photocopy this form or download it from my website, www.drlife.com. Keep the forms in a binder to monitor your progress as you move through the different levels of the Life Plan.

After each meal, write down exactly what you ate, including the calories. Also include the time that you ate and your level of hunger 20 minutes after eating, ranking it on a scale from 1 to 10. This is a good way of tracking your satiety, which can assist you in learning how to eat based upon hunger and timing rather than habit. Record how much water you drank during and before each meal so that you can add the amounts to see if you are meeting your goal. Last, you can also check off if you took your supplements each day, and list weekly which ones you are taking.

WEEK #	Monday	Tuesday	Wednesday	Thursday	Friday	Saturday	Sunday
MEAL #1							
Type:							
Time:							
Hunger level:							
Oz of water:							
MEAL #2							
Type:							
Time:							
Hunger level:							
Oz of water:							
MEAL #3							
Type:							
Time:							
Hunger level:							
Oz of water:							
MEAL #4							
Type:							
Time:							
Hunger level:							
Oz of water:							
MEAL #5							
Type:							
Time:							
Hunger level:							
Oz of water:							
Total calories:							

Mastering the Life Plan Workout Week

Now that you understand the components of the Life Plan Workout, let's put the Mighty Three pieces together to create one exercise routine that you can stick with for the long term. It's important not only to do the exercises and different types of workouts, but to do them in the right order. The following charts show exactly how this can be done.

The Life Plan combines all three modalities: flexibility and balance along with strength training, topped off with an intense cardio workout. Don't think that you've exercised by doing only one component: All three types are essential because they work synergistically so that you can have better health, a better sex life, and a better-looking body right now.

I have tried many different schedules to complete this workout. I've tried doing it all at once, and breaking out the cardio either on a different, alternating day or later in the same day that I've done my resistance training. Any way you choose will work, as long as you get all three components in as listed on the schedule. I have found that I'm best off getting my resistance training done first thing in the morning with some stretching between sets and then doing my full-blown stretching and cardio sessions in the afternoon or evening.

There are two different schedules: the first for working out at the gym; the second for working out at home. You can switch between the two for complete weeks, not one day at a time. The most important thing to remember is consistency: You'll get the best results the closer you stay to either schedule.

The Gym Workout

The gym workout is definitely more demanding on both your time and your body. Your efforts will also be apparent faster. Follow this schedule, in this order, every week. Remember that there are separate stretching/cooldown routines following both the resistance-training and cardio workouts (see Chapters 6 and 7 for details). Stick with this for at least six weeks while you are following the diet program. Once you master this schedule, you can easily move to the tougher programs featured in *The Life Plan*:

MONDAY: Resistance Training, Cardio

TUESDAY: Resistance Training, Stretching/Pilates

WEDNESDAY: Resistance Training, Cardio

THURSDAY: Resistance Training, Stretching/Pilates

FRIDAY: Resistance Training, Cardio

SATURDAY: Stretching/Pilates, Cardio (optional for beginners)

SUNDAY: Cardio (optional for beginners)

The At-Home or On-the-Road Workout

This is probably the best way to ease into a new workout routine, especially if you haven't exercised in years. Although you won't see results as quickly, don't mistake the power of this program: You'll still be getting a full-body workout. Once you master this one, you can easily move to the gym workout before taking on the tougher programs in *The Life Plan*.

This workout is also perfect for business travel if you are staying somewhere without gym access. Bands are the key to maintaining your muscle building and strength when you travel for work or vacation. They are so portable it's a no-brainer to take them with you.

This is actually an "every other day" schedule. For Week 2, continue with the recommendations for Tuesday so that you won't be performing resistance training two days in a row. Continue this rotation for at least two weeks before moving on.

MONDAY: Band Resistance Training, Cardio

TUESDAY: Stretching/Pilates, Cardio

WEDNESDAY: Band Resistance Training, Cardio

THURSDAY: Stretching/Pilates, Cardio

FRIDAY: Band Resistance Training, Cardio

SATURDAY: Stretching/Pilates, Cardio

SUNDAY: Band Resistance Training, Cardio

Life Plan Workout Journal

- -

The following chart can be photocopied or downloaded from my website, www.drlife.com. Fill in after each exercise session.

Use the "notes" section to record how you feel after each component of the workout. This way you can capture the intensity of your workout, and your energy levels before and after. Some days you may feel like you are dragging, so it's a good idea to record why you think you are not at your best. You might find that your diet is affecting your energy levels, positively or negatively. Or you might find that you are taking the stresses of the day into the gym. If lack of sleep is an issue, you should record that as well. At the beginning of each week, make sure to note the following:

- **Your weight:** Use the same scale week after week for the most accurate results.

- **Your measurements:** Measure the circumference of target areas in inches with a tape measure and record in the grid: neck, chest, arms, waist, hips, thighs, calves.

Starting Date: _____

Current Weight: _____

Measurements: Neck: Chest: Arms: Waist: Hips: Thighs: Calves:

WEEK #	Monday	Tuesday	Wednesday	Thursday	Friday	Saturday	Sunday
PILATES/ BALANCE Gym or Home: Notes:							
RESISTANCE TRAINING Gym or Home: Reps: Sets: Notes:							
CARDIO Gym or Home: Type: Time: Highest Heart Rate Achieved: Calories Burned: Notes:							

After you have kept your workout and nutrition logs for a few weeks, you can begin to analyze the information you have gathered. Try to be very objective when reading your logs and ask yourself the following questions:

1. Am I progressing? Am I losing weight, increasing muscle mass, and generally feeling better about the way I look and feel? Are my clothes fitting differently?

2. Am I working all muscle groups and at the right intensity? Am I sore after my workouts, or am I in physical pain? Do I feel it more in my arms or legs?

3. Am I resting too long between sets? Is my workout taking too long, or am I rushing through? Do I need more recovery time than what's allocated on the program?

4. Can I push myself harder? Am I tired after exercise? Am I working at my highest capability? Am I afraid of getting hurt?

5. Am I taking my supplements? Am I skipping days, or maintaining consistency?

6. Am I sleeping better at night? Do I feel rested when I wake up in the morning, and go to sleep easily at night? Do I feel energized throughout the day, or sluggish?

7. Is my flexibility better? Do I have back pain? Am I propping myself up when I have to bend to pick up something?

8. Am I eating the right amount of balanced meals?

9. Am I on track to reach my goals?

10. Am I drinking enough water?

TAKE A WORKOUT VACATION

I take one week off from cardio and resistance training every six months. This is the only time I miss workouts. This means no exercise at all for an entire week. When I return to the gym, I am really psyched and anxious, both mentally and physically, to get back at it. I'm not only energized but I know that this rest period will help prevent burnout and possible injuries due to overtraining.

Exercise with a Personal Trainer

Some men are more successful with following—and staying on—an exercise program if they have a personal trainer. Good trainers will take your training to heights you never dreamed possible. They will also prove invaluable as they:

- Teach proper form and technique

- Provide motivation

- Monitor progress

- Provide constructive criticism

- Provide positive reinforcement

- Provide an incentive (your accountability, their cost, or even better, their personality) to get to the gym

If you decide that a personal trainer would be beneficial to your exercise program, it is important that you find one who has been certified and has proven that he or she has an understanding of anatomy, exercise physiology, and exercise prescription. The top three organizations that certify personal trainers are known to offer a rigorous examination. You want your personal trainer to be certified by any one of these three:

ASK DR. LIFE

NAME: Javier R.

QUESTION: I saw you on television and I ran out and bought *The Life Plan*. I'm 52 and I've never dieted before, but I know I need to make some big changes. I'm back in the dating world and I want to look my best. Realistically, how much weight can I expect to lose per week on your program?

ANSWER: Javier, every man is different, and the amount of excess fat you're carrying, and what you've been used to eating, will determine how quickly you can get to your goal weight. You may lose a fast couple of pounds over the first few days if your old diet was filled with foods that caused inflammation and water retention. As your body adjusts to a whole new way of eating, and an increase in your metabolic rate, the pounds will continue to come off. But I don't want you to just lose body fat; I want you to be able to keep it off. A reasonable goal is dropping two to three pounds a week, but that may be tempered by an increase in muscle mass.

- NSCA: The National Strength & Conditioning Association (requires a college degree)—www.nsca-lift.org

- ACE: The American Council on Exercise—www.acefitness.org

- ACSM: The American College of Sports Medicine—www.acsm.org

• • •

You now have all the information you need to master the Life Plan in terms of your exercise and diet goals. The rest is up to you. Can you motivate yourself off the couch and into the gym? Can you find the time in even the busiest days to make change happen? For me, once I started there was no going back. I made a commitment to myself and I'm proud to say that 15 years later I still feel better every year than the year before. So for me, the choice is obvious. As I'm sure it will be for you.

Next, you'll learn the truth about male hormone replacement therapies, and the reasons you may want to consider incorporating them into your program if you suffer from true deficiencies. Most important, you'll learn how to talk intelligently about these therapies with your doctor so you can work together to determine if they are right for you.

PART THREE

MASTERING THE LIFE PLAN FOR THE REST OF YOUR LIFE

CHAPTER 9

Hormone Optimization: The Absolute Truth

I have a love-hate relationship with hormone therapies, particularly with testosterone and growth hormone. I love what they have done for me as I have learned how to correct my own deficiencies, but I hate talking about them to the uninformed, especially those in the medical community. Sometimes I feel as if I'm standing in the middle of a giant crowd completely naked, screaming the truth at the top of my lungs, yet no one is listening (actually, that might be what's needed to get their attention . . .). So once and for all, here is my all-out effort to try to get men to understand the truth about these therapies so that they can forget the myths and concentrate on the realities. Because the bottom line is this: *If you have a clinical deficiency in any particular hormone, you owe it to yourself to consider bringing up your levels so that you can prevent early, unnecessary aging and fight disease. And if you do so, you'll live a much healthier life and you won't feel old.*

Here are the facts: The loss of testosterone and other hormones that the male human body naturally produces is referred to as *andropause*. Some say it is the male equivalent to menopause, and I both agree and disagree. It's true that it refers to a hormonal loss, which is what defines menopause. But women experience a much more abrupt and obvious decline in production, and therefore many have significant symptoms as a result. For men, this hormonal decrease is slow and steady, taking place over many years, and is so subtle that you won't notice that it's happening until the day you begin to wake up and find your morning erections gone.

If you haven't heard of andropause, don't beat yourself up: Most physicians aren't familiar with the term either. In fact, andropause is not universally recognized as a disease state. As a result, men are at a real disadvantage as they begin to struggle with their own set of symptoms. Because the drop is slow and steady, symptoms of andropause are sometimes imperceptible until bigger health problems emerge. These are some of the signs that your levels are falling:

- Decreased bone density

- Decreased libido

- Loss of early morning and spontaneous erections

- Depression

- Disturbed sleep

- Emotional swings, irritability, anxiety, depression

- Fatigue

- Foggy thinking, memory lapses

- Higher body fat (especially belly fat)

- Increased cardiovascular issues

- Loss of muscle mass and strength

- Poor skin tone and saggy, wrinkled skin

- Weight gain

When your LDL and triglyceride levels are high and your HDL level is low, it's incumbent on your doctor to treat these conditions and get your levels back to healthy ranges so these abnormalities don't result in heart disease and other age-related issues. In fact, if your doctor doesn't respond to these lab values, he or she should be held accountable. And yet, when it comes to diminished hormone levels, conventional medicine doesn't accept the science. Many doctors see declining hormone levels as a natural part of aging and strongly believe that you should "just live with" these symptoms. But if you don't have to "live with" heart disease or a broken wrist, why should you have to "live with" poor health, or a lower sex drive? The answer is simple: You don't. No man needs to confront aging and its related debilitating symptoms if it is possible to reverse them, or to avoid them entirely.

Five years after winning the 1998 Body-*for*-LIFE contest, I was gaining body fat and losing strength, despite eating clean and exercising vigorously. Then I learned about Cenegenics Medical Institute and became one of their patients. After a thorough evaluation I was astonished to learn that diminished hormones could be a major part of my problem. Diagnostic blood work revealed my testosterone levels were at the bottom of the reference range. So my physician started me on testosterone therapy, and I've never looked back. Within two months I began feeling a remarkable change: more strength, better muscle mass, improved sexual function, higher energy levels, reduced cholesterol, good blood sugar control, clearer thinking, and a renewed zest for life. I know that there's no way I could accomplish all that I do today at 74 without correcting my hormone deficiencies, eating healthy, and exercising right. But that's me. You have to examine your own health issues and goals. I'm here to help you on that journey with the only thing I can give you: good advice and better science.

The best way to achieve and keep a young, lean, strong, healthy body is by making the right eating choices, exercising intelligently and consistently, and correcting hormonal deficiencies. Healthy aging physicians like me use this three-pronged approach to achieve superior health outcomes with our patients. Not only does this approach make it possible to avoid premature disability and death, but energy levels (including sexual energy), lean muscle mass, bone density, and cognitive function also improve. An additional benefit is that the immune system is strengthened, which can help you remain disease-free as long as possible.

TESTOSTERONE AND SEX

Decreased libido and erectile quality are the symptoms most frequently associated with falling testosterone levels, yet they are actually some of the latest symptoms, with other symptoms present much sooner.

The Truth about Testosterone

What else do I need to say: You can't have decent sex without testosterone. Testosterone is commonly thought of as the driving force that makes men macho, but it is really much more than that: It's one of the most critical aspects of your overall health. It's very necessary for maintaining high energy levels and vitality, increasing your muscle mass and overall strength (men simply can't build muscle without it), enhancing your ability to burn body fat (especially around the waist and inside the abdomen), improving your mood and emotional well-being, preventing bone loss, keeping your mind sharp, and protecting your heart.

From age 30 onward, testosterone begins to drop 1 to 3 percent annually. Low blood testosterone levels can also occur in younger men—in fact it is now estimated that 20 million American men of all ages suffer from what is called low testosterone syndrome. This includes 2 to 3 percent of men in their twenties, 20 to 30 percent in their thirties and forties, on up to well over 50 percent of men in their sixties and seventies. This means that by the time you've reached your midforties, if you haven't started complaining that you are feeling older, you will soon.

This sense of "feeling older" may present itself as declining work productivity, a desire to take a nap Saturday afternoons, or telling your spouse or partner that you're too tired to have sex. Your once-effective workout won't deliver the same results, and you might start gaining weight. You might be annoyed by the younger guys in the office who can party all night long and still get the job done during the day. And all this may be affecting your mood and your relationships.

The Truth: Stress Shuts Down Testosterone Production

An important and often overlooked cause of decreased testosterone levels is emotional stress. Hundreds of thousands of years ago the "fight or flight" alarm reaction system possessed by our ancestors served as a major survival mechanism for very short-lived life-or-death situations. This system releases stress hormones with high catabolic activity, enabling our predecessors to rapidly break down body stores of fat and muscle for immediate energy that was essential for their survival.

We have all inherited this same genetic code. Worse, the stress we encounter is prolonged, cumulative, and often chronic: bad job, bad marriage, financial worries, global warming, to name a few. This results in the continued release of stress hormones, which severely inhibits testosterone production and may be the greatest underlying cause of aging and the development of degenerative diseases such as heart disease and arthritis. That's why it is very important not only to keep testosterone levels high, but also to do your best to minimize stress.

For me, the best way I've found to do this is through exercise. When I'm in that zone I can forget everything else around me. That's why I never complain that I "have to" work out for an hour a day or more: It's my release from the rest of the world and from my own problems.

If you find that you are turning to alcohol, prescription or street drugs, or food to release the tension of the day, I strongly suggest that you rethink these choices and seek professional help if you need it. There is definitely a better way to relieve your stress.

The Truth: Low Testosterone Affects Your Health beyond Your Penis

Testosterone is an anabolic, or tissue-building, hormone. A man with low testosterone could face greater risk for heart disease, Alzheimer's, prostate cancer, frailty, and sarcopenia.

Men with low testosterone have a 33 percent greater death risk over their next 18 years of life compared with men having higher testosterone.

The heart—and not the testicles—is the organ with the highest concentration of testosterone receptors. Testosterone is associated with several positive effects on cardiac health. It has been linked with reducing coronary artery disease (CAD) and hypertension risks as well as with improving cardiac function in patients with preexisting heart disease. In large population studies it has been found that low testosterone levels are associated with increased risk of atherosclerotic cardiac disease. Older men treated with testosterone can show decreases in total cholesterol and LDL. Low testosterone levels also are correlated with a greater degree of atherosclerotic blockage when coronary artery disease is present.

The brain is second only to the heart in terms of abundance of testosterone receptors. Testosterone is associated with maintaining cognitive function, lowered dementia risk, and decreasing symptoms of depression, anxiety, and panic disorders. Maintaining testosterone levels carries a significant cognitive benefit.

Testosterone is also the key to fighting inflammation. Recent research from Friedrich Schiller University in Germany revealed an intriguing fact: Men and women do not respond to inflammatory stimuli in the same manner. It turns out that the enzyme phospholipase D—an inflammatory stimulus and regulator of critical aspects of cell physiology—is not as active in male cells as it is in female cells. Based on that, the study suggests that testosterone is pivotal to maintaining a proper immune response and protecting the body from inflammation. This is important because inflammation is the underlying cause of most chronic diseases related to aging.

Diminished hormones, particularly testosterone, put men at risk for debilitating conditions, such as hip fractures. In addition to testosterone's correlation with declining bone density, it is also linked intimately with muscle loss. Studies have looked at the relationship between testosterone replacement and a return to a more favorable body composition. The consensus from the medical literature is that testosterone supplementation is accompanied by gains in lean mass across all age groups. It is associated with reduced body fat, with some preferential fat loss seen in the abdomen.

Although abuse of testosterone is linked with increased risk of cardiovascular disease and sudden death, higher testosterone levels within the normal range of a 35- to 40-year-old have been found to be associated with a more favorable cardiovascular profile. So when I'm asked whether the medical community should consider including testosterone measurements in the evaluation of male patients, I say "yes," and even take it a step further to recommend treatment.

The Myth: Testosterone Alone Can Fix ED

An estimated 34 percent of all American men ages 40–70 suffer from some significant level of ED (erectile dysfunction). An August 2008 study demonstrated that Metabolic Syndrome's elements, which include obesity (especially abdominal obesity), diabetes, high blood pressure, and cholesterol problems, have a common denominator: testosterone deficiency. But this does not mean that by correcting testosterone levels you'll be back in the saddle.

Erectile dysfunction can be an early warning sign of underlying vascular disease and diabetes. Research reveals that many men experience erectile dysfunction four to five years before having a heart attack. Other studies from the Mayo Clinic show that men with ED have an 80 percent higher risk for coronary artery disease. This means that not only do you have to correct your testosterone levels, but you also have to have your risk for heart disease evaluated and start on a preventive program that lowers your risk for diabetes and progressive vascular disease, which may lead to a heart attack or stroke. Might I suggest you try the Life Plan?

Therapies that restore natural testosterone levels show real improvement on several sexual performance fronts. In studies of sexual function, mood, and well-being, testosterone supplementation correlated with improved quality of life. That should be no surprise: What man would not be having more sex if he was in a better mood? So don't get trapped in the denial game. Talk to your doctor if you're having issues with sexual function, not only to regain your intimate life and self-esteem, but also to improve your overall health.

The Truth: There Is No Link between Elevated Testosterone Levels and Prostate Cancer

Most physicians I meet have it all wrong when it comes to prostate cancer and testosterone. While testosterone is associated with prostate cancer risk, it is in the exact opposite relationship than they believe. Historically, doctors feared that raising testosterone levels may cause existing prostate cancer to grow. This fear stems from a 1941 journal article reporting that testosterone injections caused an enhanced rate of prostate growth and castration caused prostate regression. Unfortunately, this study was conducted on one patient. Further science since then, however, has failed to support this review. A large longitudinal study found no relationship between testosterone concentrations and the risk for prostate cancer, except to find that one risk factor of prostate cancer was low testosterone levels, not high.

The Truth: Testosterone Therapies Are Safe and Effective

Supplementing testosterone has been historically discouraged by most of the medical community. But fortunately, times are changing. Since *The Life Plan* came out, I've been featured in articles from the *New York Times* to *Esquire*. Some of the feedback has been less than complimentary, but I don't care. I have a choice about how I'm going to manage my health, and so do you. You can choose to grow old and weak, or you can choose to do something about it. Doctors continue to report that reversing hormone deficiencies is unsafe and, more to the point, "unnatural." I don't think that there is anything unnatural about maintaining a younger, healthier, more vibrant body and lifestyle.

In terms of safety, the pharmaceutical industry has realized that testosterone therapy is big business, and has responded to increased demand by developing new methods for administering natural testosterone. Side effects are rare and typically occur during the first few months, but usually resolve themselves. These can include skin reactions such as acne, oily skin, erythema, breast tenderness, erythrocytosis (increased production of red blood cells), COPD (chronic obstructive pulmonary disease), sleep apnea, and lower-extremity edema (swelling).

There are many different ways to administer testosterone. These are the most popular:

- **Transdermal:** Gels, creams, or patches. I'm not a fan of this approach. Its absorption can be affected by weather conditions and it can be transferred to your partner, or even your kids. Plus, you need to apply it daily.

- **Pellets:** Surgically implanted into your muscles. This testosterone delivery method slowly leaks into your system as it dissolves over a period of weeks. Problems arise if levels become too high; you'll need to have a pellet taken out. Low levels mean another pellet needs to be inserted.

- **Injections in the upper outer buttocks or upper outer thigh:** This is my preferred method. Testosterone injected into the muscle once a week results in creating a steady state of this hormone in your bloodstream, which in turn maximizes the health benefits of testosterone replacement therapy. I teach my patients how to give themselves this injection and most have no problem with it.

- **Under the Tongue** (twice daily): This method of testosterone administration has not been studied well and carries with it a potential risk of serious side effects.

ASK DR. LIFE

NAME: Dwight B.

QUESTION: I have your book and it is great. I've been on bio-identical testosterone for several years. Due to low free levels my physician has just put me on injections every two weeks. If I want to change to weekly to maintain more consistent levels, do I just cut my dose in half? Do you have a schedule, strength, and volume you can share? Thanks, Dwight.

ANSWER: Dwight, talk to your doctor about putting you on a once-a-week regimen that will halve your biweekly dose. I typically start my patients on 0.5 cc of testosterone cypionate (200 mg/cc) intramuscular injection every week in the upper lateral thigh.

The Truth: You Can Increase Testosterone Naturally

Before you rush out to your doctor's office to determine if you have a deficiency, there are a few very important things you need to know. Testosterone replacement therapy may not be necessary for every man, because many of you can achieve the same results naturally by changing your lifestyle. There are many things you can do to increase your levels of testosterone without the help of the pharmaceutical industry.

The first is improving your eating habits by following the Life Plan. Studies clearly show that low-fat diets result in low testosterone levels, and diets higher in protein, lower in carbohydrates, and moderate in fats result in the greatest sustained high levels of testosterone. As I've said, men must eat plenty of lean protein, because it stimulates the hormone glucagon and other muscle-building responses important for increased testosterone release. Eating more vegetables and nontropical fruit and limiting the intake of simple sugars and starches (high-glycemic-index carbs) will help, as this type of low-glycemic diet lowers the hormones insulin and cortisol, which not only make you bloated but interfere with testosterone production. The essential fatty acids (omega 3s) found in fish and flaxseed, which we discussed earlier, are essential for the body to produce testosterone.

When it comes to increasing your own production of testosterone, the next area to look at is exercise. Both a lack of physical activity and excessive physical activity (overtraining) will decrease your testosterone level. Testosterone actually diminishes during extended periods of endurance training. After 60 minutes of exercise, cortisol levels begin to rise and testosterone levels decrease as a result of overtraining. This reduction can last up to six days!

Testosterone levels increase the most when an exercise program is short and very intense. It's the core exercises, such as squats and bench presses, that train large muscle groups and that do the best job of raising testosterone. For this reason, some men who follow my program split their training sessions up and don't perform aerobic training during the same session that they lift weights. If your testosterone levels are not an issue, then you don't have to worry about splitting your training.

Last, make sure you get a full eight hours of sleep as often as possible to maximize your testosterone production. Hormone production is greatest when your body is at rest, which is why it's important to get plenty of good sleep.

NAME: Michael M.

QUESTION: I love your work and I have a tremendous amount of respect for your work in antiaging. Your latest book is fantastic. I am a 57 endurance athlete. Last July I was diagnosed with a deep vein thrombosis (DVT) in my right calf. I have been taking AndroGel for 7 years, 6–9 months out of the year. Testosterone level 800 approx. Since my diagnosis, my doctor has taken me off the AndroGel. My question for you: Can I resume AndroGel at some point or is supplemental testosterone therapy contraindicated for someone with a blood clot? All blood tests negative for genetic, biochemical clotting, and I don't have a family history of clotting. Not being able to take testosterone would be a real loss for me.

ANSWER: Michael, first I would need to know why you developed a blood clot in your leg. It is very unusual for a guy your age who is as active as you are to have a DVT. Second, I'm not a fan of transdermal formulations of testosterone, but I doubt that it played a part in your developing a blood clot. I much prefer testosterone that is injected once weekly. Because testosterone therapies are perfectly calibrated to each individual, I would recommend seeing a hematologist—a blood specialist—and get his or her opinion before resuming testosterone replacement therapy.

The Reality: When Should I Start Testosterone Therapy?

You need to work with your current physician to come up with a program that optimizes your hormone levels. The first step is to obtain the proper testing, which I've outlined in Chapter 10. In terms of testosterone, a total serum testosterone test done first thing in the morning is necessary to determine your current levels. Some specialists, including myself, believe that you also need a free or unbound testosterone-level check.

If you have borderline or even very low testosterone levels, you can first try to raise your levels through exercise, weight loss, proper nutrition, supplementation, avoiding smoking, minimizing the use of alcohol, improving sleep, and controlling the stress in your life before going on testosterone therapy. Get rid of excess body fat, especially around your belly, since this elevates your estrogen levels, which compete with testosterone receptors throughout your body. Make sure you don't lose body fat too fast (more than two pounds per week), because if your body thinks you are starving, testosterone levels will plummet and your muscles will shrink.

If all of these efforts fail to restore your healthy levels of testosterone, then find a doctor knowledgeable in treating andropause who can help you. You will need to have your bloodwork monitored every three to four months to make sure target levels of total and free testosterone have been reached and not exceeded. At my office, every man undergoes a highly comprehensive evaluation to first determine if a clinical hormone deficiency exists. Any man needing a correction of hormone deficiencies has bloodwork done at six weeks, and again every three to four months after that to ensure levels stay in the healthy range.

Because every man's hormone levels are unique, it's impossible to know exactly how high your levels were before they declined. What's more, not every man is a good candidate for testosterone therapy. Discuss your current health status with your doctor, especially if you have a history of obstructive sleep apnea or heart failure. If you have either of these you need to see an appropriate specialist before starting therapy. Most men require some fine-tuning of their treatments until the best results are achieved. You should notice that your symptoms begin to improve in three to six weeks after you start treatment.

The Truth about Growth Hormone

I also have strong feelings about human growth hormone therapies because I have witnessed remarkable reversals in aging and disease by using them myself. Unfortunately, the medical community and the media continue to get this one all wrong. I also want to make it very clear that as with any type of medicine, growth hormone should not be abused, and it should be used only when it is determined to be absolutely necessary—that is, for treating a documented deficiency.

Human growth hormone is naturally produced by the pituitary gland in the brain and is critical for repair throughout your body. Its ability to reverse many of the major effects of aging, including muscle loss, weakness, skin tone and texture, excess body fat deposits, energy depletion, and declining immune function, is unparalleled in today's medicine. It can also help boost your sex drive as well as sexual potency.

Healthy aging physicians like me have embraced human growth hormone (hGH) as a treatment option for adults with clinical proven deficiencies. It was first developed to aid in growth for children of small stature, and it is still prescribed for this purpose by endocrinologists. Before 1986, human growth hormone was harvested from cadavers and carried a risk for transmission of disease to its recipients. Since then, growth hormone has been commercially produced in laboratories by major pharmaceutical firms, and issues concerning disease transmission are no longer applicable: The supply of hGH is safe, available, and easy to administer.

Just as with unregulated testosterone use, we know that some athletes abuse this treatment when they take hGH to increase strength and improve their performance. It's important to know that hGH treatments are completely legal if you're diagnosed as being deficient and an FDA-approved formulation is obtained with a doctor's prescription after appropriate clinical testing proves your deficiency. However, it's unclear whether it actually does improve your athletic prowess. We do know that it will allow you to recover from injury faster, but only if you have a deficiency.

As we age, our growth hormone production decreases. Adult hGH levels decline by half from ages 20 to 60, and the loss accelerates thereafter. Yet the typical decline begins at age 40, meaning that it is highly unlikely that a 20- to 35-year-old athlete will have a growth hormone deficiency. If he did, these would be the telltale symptoms:

- Decreased libido

- Decreased muscular strength

- Depression

- Diabetes

- Dyslipidemia (abnormal cholesterol panel)

- Endothelial dysfunction

- Fatigue

- Hypertension

- Hypothyroidism

- Memory loss

- Metabolic Syndrome

- Obesity (especially abdominal obesity)

- Osteoporosis

- Poor cognitive stability

- Reduced exercise capacity

- Sarcopenia

- Sleep apnea

- Sleep disturbance

The Truth: Growth Hormone Assists Repair throughout the Body

Growth hormone (Somatotropin) is a protein-based polypeptide hormone secreted by the anterior pituitary gland in your brain. It stimulates cellular growth, reproduction, and regeneration. Today somatotropin can be synthesized through recombinant DNA technology and is abbreviated as "hGH." Mounting evidence shows that adults with a somatotropin deficiency have impaired health, which then improves with hGH replacement therapy.

The following diseases are related to growth hormone deficiency:

- **Cardiovascular disease:** Growth hormone protects against endothelial dysfunction, atherosclerotic plaque development, Metabolic Syndrome, plaque instability, and ischemic heart disease. Low levels are now considered to represent an additional independent risk factor for cardiovascular disease.

- **Stroke:** Low levels of circulating growth hormone are a predictor of stroke and the severity of stroke.

- **Obesity:** The health risks associated with obesity are closely correlated with abdominal or visceral fat. Visceral fat causes Metabolic Syndrome, which is associated with serious metabolic disorders, including inflammation, heart disease, cancer, stroke, insulin resistance, diabetes, and Alzheimer's disease. Visceral fat is associated with a decrease in normal growth hormone levels as well as its distribution. Numerous studies of growth hormone replacement therapy have found that this form of treatment decreases fat mass and increases lean body mass.

The Truth: hGH Is Expensive

- -

Human growth hormone therapies can run as much as $1,500/month, and in most cases are not covered by typical health insurance policies. However, the costs of treating the diseases associated with untreated growth hormone deficiency over your lifetime far outweigh this expense.

Myth: Growth Hormone Therapy May Increase Cancer Risk

- -

Current clinical guidelines from the Endocrine Society state that there is no evidence that the incidence of tumors is increased by growth hormone therapy, even though some of the media have clung to this as a potential risk factor. In 2001, the Growth Hormone Research Society extensively reviewed the question of whether growth hormone therapy is associated with tumor growth. Their final statement was clear: For patients receiving growth hormone therapy, "No additional monitoring for other malignant tumors (such as tumors of the prostate, breast, or colon) is currently suggested beyond the accepted standard of care for the patient's age and sex."

The Truth: You Must Test to Determine a Deficiency

- -

Doctors like me who administer growth hormone must adhere to state and federal guidelines. First, every doctor must conduct the appropriate testing required before administering this treatment to make sure that there is a clinical deficiency. The gold standard for diagnosing a growth hormone deficiency has been the insulin tolerance test (ITT): It is a stimulation test used by many endocrinologists. Another stimulation test is the glucagon stimulation test, which is considered much safer than the ITT. Many investigators and clinicians reject the ITT and other stimulation tests for diagnosing adult growth hormone deficiency and rely on a blood test called IGF-1 (Insulin-like Growth Factor-1) as a more reliable diagnostic and therapeutic marker of growth hormone deficiency.

In spite of all this controversy, the FDA and hGH manufacturers have maintained their positions that stimulation testing is necessary and required for an accurate diagnosis. In my practice, I use glucagon pituitary stimulation testing as a prerequisite for diagnosing growth hormone deficiency. Once therapy begins, all of my patients receiving hGH must be followed closely with repeat blood draws every four to five months to ensure that their levels are in the correct range and markers of disease are improving.

The Truth: You Can Improve Your Production of Growth Hormone Naturally

As with testosterone, you can increase your own production of growth hormone through the correction of other hormone deficiencies, and by following a comprehensive program such as the Life Plan, which maximizes diet and requires significant exercise. I'm pleased when my patients follow my protocol and come back to my office after just eight weeks with significant increases in their growth hormone levels. Once your body learns to do this, it will continue increased production as you continue the program.

Exercise can play a significant role in growth hormone secretion. About 10–20 minutes of aerobic exercise causes a rise in serum levels that peak at the end of that period and is sustained for up to two hours. If you train at 85 percent or more of your target HR_{max} for 20 to 25 minutes, you will stimulate your pituitary gland to produce more growth hormone. The same applies to lifting heavy weights that involve large muscle groups. These exercises include squats, dead lifts, and bench presses.

If you were looking for the proverbial "last straw" in order to stop bad eating habits, it's been well documented that a high-saturated-fat, high-glycemic diet reduces growth hormone secretion by 30 percent. Yet following a low-glycemic diet high in lean proteins and healthy fats can increase your levels. Amino acids such as arginine, found in all protein sources, stimulate growth hormone secretion. Positive correlations have also been shown between growth hormone production and the intake of micronutrients such as calcium, iron, potassium, magnesium, niacin, phosphorus, riboflavin, thiamine, and zinc, found in vegetables, fruits, and nutraceuticals. While the Life Plan Diets were initially developed for heart health, the growth hormone benefits are equally important.

We produce growth hormone all day long, but mostly during deep sleep. Men who don't sleep well or don't sleep enough will invariably have low levels of growth hormone, and many will be growth hormone deficient. This is one more reason why getting proper sleep is an absolute must while you are following the Life Plan.

If you follow the Life Plan for eight weeks and your growth hormone levels remain low and the signs and symptoms have not improved, I would suggest that you undergo a stimulation test to confirm your suspicions of growth hormone deficiency and comply with the FDA requirements for a complete diagnosis of adult-onset growth hormone deficiency.

The Reality: When Should I Start Hormone Therapy?

You need to work with your physician to come up with a program that optimizes all of your hormone levels: You can't just pick and choose which ones you want to work on. The first step is to obtain the proper evaluation and testing, which I've outlined in Chapter 10. It is essential that you find a physician who is knowledgeable about the diagnosis and treatment of hormone deficiencies. He or she needs to be fully informed about the vital role the right kind of exercise and nutrition play in overall health and longevity. He or she needs to be totally up to speed with the early diagnosis of heart disease and how to treat all of the inflammatory risk factors.

Not every man is a good candidate for testosterone therapy. Discuss your current health status with your doctor, especially if you have a history of obstructive sleep apnea or heart failure. If you have any of these, you need to see an appropriate specialist before starting therapy.

Other Hormones to Consider

There is a wide range of hormones that you can consider replacing, depending on your current health status and deficiencies you may have. However, not all hormone therapies are the same. Synthetic hormones like methyltestosterone carry a black box warning connecting them to liver cancer. It has also been shown that growth hormones harvested from cadavers cause cancer.

I prescribe only pharmaceutically approved hormones, which are plant-based, natural, and safe. These hormones produce the same physiological responses as the body's own natural hormones. I commonly prescribe for men the following:

- **DHEA (Dehydroepiandrosterone):** Produced in the adrenal cortex of the adrenal gland as well as the testicles, it is then converted to estrogen and testosterone. Reestablishing DHEA balance to more youthful levels can enhance sexual desire, performance, and overall mood. It is also used for increasing production of testosterone and growth hormone, as well as combating chronic fatigue syndrome, depression, memory loss, and osteoporosis. DHEA is so mild that it can be purchased over the counter as a supplement, but I recommend pharmaceutical-grade DHEA to make sure you are really getting what you are paying for. I have tested many of my patients taking inferior DHEA products and found, not surprisingly, low blood levels.

- **Thyroid (T3 and/or T4):** Some men experiencing sexual dysfunction may actually have underlying thyroid disease. When we correct these deficiencies, they not only feel better, but they perform better in bed. These hormones can also help relieve depression, brain fog, fatigue, and other age-related symptoms. Thyroid hormone therapies can be obtained only with a doctor's prescription.

- **Melatonin:** Supplementing with melatonin helps regulate sleep patterns, but it also has antioxidant properties for overall health and protection from cancer. Melatonin can help you relax, so it may also improve sexual performance. This can be purchased over the counter as a supplement. It has a short half-life of only two or three hours, so I recommend sustained-release formulations.

CHAPTER 10

The Life Plan and Your Doctor

The three prongs of the Life Plan—diet, exercise, and correcting hormone imbalances—will absolutely put you on a pathway to better health. They work synergistically to control aging, reverse existing disease, and prevent future illness. However, some of us may already be facing health issues that need to be addressed now, before you start this program. This chapter is meant to go over some of the most frequent medical concerns that men face; the ones I see in my office every day. Some definitely fall into the "sensitive topics" category, and it might be painful for you to think about resolving them. But you must be man enough to take control of your health, and that might mean facing some of your demons or coming to grips with disappointment.

Addiction and the Type A Personality

The men who come into my office are typically very driven individuals. They are high achievers—Type A personalities—and often they are workaholics. They can't seem to slow down, and frankly, they don't want to. They just don't want to get old.

While this mind-set might sound appealing, especially if you are the type who constantly seems to be stuck in a rut, the truth is, this go-go lifestyle can be a sign of a deeper problem.

That's because in one way or another, some of these men are struggling with an addiction. They may be either addicted to their career or addicted to money and "stuff" in general, or I may discover during the examination that they are addicted to sex, drugs, alcohol, cigarettes, and very often, food. I don't pass judgment on these men, because I know that these addictions are not their fault: Their brain chemistry is what drives them to this type of behavior. And better still, I know that these men can be helped.

The answers are found in a fuller understanding of the brain. The intersection between personality and health resides in your head, because the brain controls every decision you make. Its chemical messengers—called neurotransmitters—are constantly relaying signals from different parts of the brain to the body, telling us when to eat, when to sleep, how to move, and how to respond to stimuli. These messengers are also responsible for how different things make us feel, from fatty foods and exercise to vodka, gambling, drugs, and even generosity.

The neurotransmitter dopamine is released by the brain's neurons and delivered to its receptors every time you are exposed to something that excites you. The way you respond to the stimulus is determined by how much dopamine is actually released. For example, experiences that cause dopamine to be activated will be decoded as pleasurable: In a sense, the dopamine you are receiving is like a reward. And if you are the type of person who responds to pleasure, you will do anything you can to make that experience occur again and again. This is the potential beginning of any addictive cycle.

What can happen next is the downside: Each time you are exposed to the same thing that turned you on, you need more dopamine to achieve that "rush." But in order to produce more dopamine, you need more of the stimuli. So if your big dopamine trigger is alcohol, one drink won't do it the second time around. Instead, each subsequent time you need more and more alcohol to achieve a full dopamine hit, which creates that sense of excitement or pleasure. This is why I know that addicts—no matter what their vice—are for the most part just regular people who are responding to instructions from their physical brain to seek out and score whatever it is that will release the most dopamine. Now let's see what this might mean for you.

Addiction Part 1: Food

For many of us, food is an easy, natural reward. We've been taught to celebrate any "job well done" with a good meal or special dessert. And many of us also know that it's hard to have just one cookie or potato chip. Before we used to call that a lack of willpower, but now science knows better. Research from a June 2006 study published in the *Journal of Neuroscience* showed that the more people ate, the less dopamine was released: This makes us eat more of whatever we crave to get that full dopamine hit, just as I described above. However, the desire for a particular food, or what we refer to as cravings, signals the release of dopamine, which is why any type of craving is a fundamental component of addiction. In a 2005 landmark study, Drs. Nora Volkow and Roy Wise determined that the brain responded to food in the same way it responds to heavily addictive drugs like cocaine. If you experience food cravings and find that you need more of a particular food each time you eat it in order to feel satisfied, you may be addicted to food.

Chronic exposure to foods high in combinations of sugar, fat, and salt can rewire the brain to promote and amplify this craving mechanism. Earlier in the book we talked about the powerful nature of sugar in terms of food addiction. Today's American diet is primarily made up of carbohydrates, and as much as 75 percent of us overreact to carbs by producing too much insulin, leading directly to Type 2 diabetes. Fatty foods are a second problem. Dr. Ann Kelly from the University of Wisconsin authored a study showing that fat is highly addictive, especially when you add sugar or salt to it. Just thinking about this research makes me think of—and want to eat—ice cream!

Some of us may be genetically predisposed to reduced dopamine levels, making us even more susceptible to overconsumption/addictive behavior. But there's hope. You can rewire your circuitry and reboot your brain as I did to beat addiction and feel better than ever.

First, review these signs and symptoms to determine if you may have a food addiction. If you answer "true" to more than four of them, discuss the outcome with your doctor, as well as the specific issues that triggered your positive response.

1. When food, eating, or my weight are the topics of discussion, I withdraw or attempt to change the subject. T/F

2. There is at least one type of food I must eat every day. T/F

3. I use food as a way to deal with my emotions. T/F

4. I often eat in front of the TV, or graze mindlessly throughout the day. T/F

5. I spend time every day buying food for myself or my family. T/F

6. I know I eat far more than I need of certain foods, but it makes me feel better to eat it, even when I'm not hungry. T/F

7. I feel powerless when I have a craving. T/F

8. I often feel sluggish after I eat. T/F

9. I can't go to bed without having a late-night sweet snack. T/F

10. My favorite foods include doughnuts, ice cream, French fries, cookies, breakfast cereals, or chips. T/F

An Addiction Pushes an Epidemic

Today, over a third of U.S. adults are obese. I believe that food addiction could be the number-one culprit behind America's obesity epidemic, as the American diet over the past 30 years has been overrun by salty, high-sugar, high-glycemic carbs. Before the 1980s, only about 13 percent of Americans were considered to be obese. By the end of that decade more than 21 percent of the U.S. adult population was overweight or obese. Ironically, this epidemic began at the same time that the federal government was recommending that we follow a low-fat diet.

At that time, fat was considered the main offender behind a growing trend of increased rates of heart disease. Food manufacturers stepped up to the plate (literally) and started promoting low-fat foods, replacing many of our favorite meals with carbohydrate-dense ones: Gone was steak, in came pasta. Today, the average American adult consumes 60 more pounds of processed grains each year than he or she did in the 1970s. We're also consuming 30 percent more of the natural and artificial sweeteners that are found in almost all packaged goods. This has led people to increase their caloric intake by more than 400 calories a day.

In 1992, the U.S. government came up with another great idea: the food pyramid. This was supposed to help us make better food choices. Yet even though the data were there, our government missed the forest for the trees. The link between diseases, early death, and over-indulgence in sugar and high-glycemic carbohydrates was ignored, and the government created a food program in which the biggest portion of every meal remained carbohydrates.

The problem was, and still is, glycation, which is what the body does as it digests high-glycemic carbohydrates. You can think of insulin as a switch. When you start eating foods that increase blood sugars and glycation, the insulin switch turns on, and your body has the ability to process the sugar into energy. However, when there is an excess amount of sugar, the insulin switch doesn't function effectively, and the extra sugars are turned into and stored as body fat. When the insulin switch is turned off after you've eaten, then the body can tap into its fat stores for energy. But if you keep eating high-glycemic foods, the insulin switch never turns off. This causes your blood sugar and insulin levels to remain elevated and sets the stage for Type 2 diabetes. Over 16 million Americans have this form of diabetes and half of them don't even know it. Type 2 diabetes mostly occurs in people over age 40, but today we are seeing more and more of this devastating disease in children and adolescents.

When we change our diet to remove sugar and other high-glycemic foods, as I've described earlier in the book, you can add as many as 10–15 years to your life and avoid or reverse Type 2 diabetes and its related diseases, including Metabolic Syndrome and heart disease. And with the proper exercise program, those won't be additional nursing home years. They'll be active, vibrant years of great health.

ASK DR. LIFE

NAME: Stewart R.

QUESTION: I'm 56 and I just learned that I have Type 2 diabetes. How is this going to affect my lifestyle?

ANSWER: Stewart, you're going to have to start thinking about food in a whole new way. Focus on an eating program just like the Life Plan: Every meal needs to feature low-glycemic carbs with a portion of protein, and you need to eat this way five times a day. Exercise is also critical. Regular workouts affect glucose and insulin levels so that they can return to a more normal state. Talk to your doctor, and together you can create a program—or use mine as a starting point—while you learn to monitor your glucose levels to prevent your diabetes from pushing other chronic diseases into the picture.

DIABETES AFFECTS YOUR SEX LIFE

- 58 percent of men with diabetes report having erectile dysfunction (ED).

- Diabetic men are three times more likely to have ED than nondiabetics.

Addiction Part 2: Alcohol, Prescription Drugs, and More

It's very possible that food is not your vice, or maybe not your only vice. You might have issues with alcohol, prescription drugs, street drugs, cigarettes, or gambling. Or it may be something else entirely: hoarding (or as some call it, "collecting"), sex, whatever. It truly doesn't matter what your drug of choice is, because the fix is the same. Men all across the country are dealing with these same problems, and they need medical attention. I also know that with the proper care, which may include medications and counseling, most men can beat their addictions and reverse their downhill path to early death.

The Life Plan Addiction Quiz

Review these questions just as before. These are geared to addictive behavior in general. If you answer "true" to more than four of them, seek help, and talk about your specific issue with a health professional. Don't hesitate to get help because you are embarrassed; I can guarantee that any doctor or therapist you see has heard it all before.

1. A doctor has told me that my addiction has related health issues, yet I haven't stopped. T/F

2. My friends or family have talked to me about how my behavior is negatively affecting their lives. T/F

3. I often have anxiety, sweating, shakes, or feel sick. T/F

4. I shop in different liquor stores to avoid being recognized at any one store. T/F

5. I spend a great deal of time getting my buzz going. T/F

6. Most people don't understand me. T/F

7. I feel like I have a secret life. T/F

8. All my life I've been the victim of circumstances. T/F

9. I avoid family functions. T/F

10. I have a hard time getting up in the morning. T/F

The Way to Break Addictive Behaviors

The first step in successfully dealing with addictive behaviors is to recognize that you have them. When you can determine which foods, substances, or behaviors are addicting for you, then treat them like heroin—something that you know is especially dangerous—and completely avoid them.

Overcoming an addiction is hard work. I know that it takes time, persistence, and a single-minded approach. There is no such thing as a "free day" when it comes to avoiding these foods or behaviors. It takes about a week of strict avoidance before cravings go away, and it may feel like the longest week of your life. But once the cravings are gone you will never have to worry about them again—unless you go back.

I know that I'm a Type A personality, and there's not much I can do to change that. However, I have been able to change my behaviors: how I deal with people and my own inner demons. Over the past 15 years I have had great success in controlling my own destructive addictions—food and alcohol. My secret has been to replace them with what I consider healthy addictions (exercise, clean eating, music, massage, stress-reduction strategies, and so on). Not every day has been perfect, and the journey has not always been easy. However, I'm much better off today than I was for the majority of my life, and I know that if I can master my addictions, so can you.

Heart Disease

When I say that cardiovascular disease is the number-one killer of men, I really mean it. Even with the best medicine has to offer, 65 percent of American men will still die as a result of it. Worse, 35 to 50 percent of those cardiac deaths are considered "sudden and unexpected." That means that most men are not fully aware of their health status, because with the right preventive treatments, you can keep cardiac diseases, including stroke, at bay.

One of the hardest concepts for men to swallow is that they must find the time to see their doctor once a year. I can't stress this enough, especially when it comes to your heart. Here's why: Cardiac disease starts in your twenties, and possibly as far back as your preteens. And over 90 percent of heart attack events occur at arterial sites undetectable with conventional diagnostics (such as stress testing). So if you are seeing your doctor annually and your doctor is tuned in to detecting the earliest signs of vascular disease, you're much more likely to make the lifestyle changes that can keep you in good health for a very long time and help you avoid a heart attack or stroke. This is why I believe, and the medical literature supports me, that the better preventive care your heart gets—including the right exercise, nutrition, nutraceuticals, healthy hormone levels, and state-of-the-art, annual bloodwork—the easier it is to eliminate the causes of heart disease now, and for years to come.

My approach, which I urge you to share with your doctor, is centered on proactively protecting your endothelium, the thin, one-cell layer lining the interior of your heart and entire vascular tree (arteries and veins). The endothelium forms a dynamic interface between your blood and your body. Endothelial cells are important for many reasons. They secrete substances—like the vitally important messenger molecule nitric oxide—that regulate homeostasis, keep blood moving smoothly, control blood pressure, ensure vascular tone, control inflammatory processes, and prevent oxidation and coagulation. When not properly cared for, your endothelial cells can become dysfunctional, putting you at risk for numerous disease processes that cause atherosclerosis, hypertension, inflammatory syndromes, heart disease, stroke, and dementia. A 2003 Mayo Clinic paper defined endothelial dysfunction as the "ultimate risk" among all the cardiovascular risk factors. If you have any of the conditions/ histories listed below, you must start working with your doctor to improve the health of your endothelium. And the first step will be to continue following the Life Plan:

- Family history of heart disease and/or confirmed heart disease, based on carotid ultrasound diagnostics, abnormal stress test, or an elevated coronary calcium score

- History of elevated LDL levels or low HDL levels

- Elevated total cholesterol levels

- Metabolic Syndrome

- Elevated triglyceride levels

- Elevated cardio CRP levels

- Evidence of vascular disease

The Deadly Myths of Heart Disease

- **Cholesterol causes heart attacks:** The fact is that 50 percent of men who suffer from heart attacks have normal cholesterol. It's true that overabundant LDL particles can accumulate in the walls of your arteries—forming plaque. This is called atherosclerosis. However, arterial wall inflammation is what triggers a heart attack, not the plaque. Inflammation can cause a rupture or erosion of the plaque, which immediately causes a blood clot to form in the artery, leading to a heart attack or stroke. The secret to preventing heart attacks and strokes is not only to prevent plaque buildup, but also to eliminate inflammation with the right kind of diet, smart exercise, supplements, and correcting hormonal deficiencies—in other words, the Life Plan.

- **HDL is "good" cholesterol:** A 2012 study jointly published by MIT and Harvard researchers casts doubt on the true value of "good cholesterol." This study makes use of powerful databases of genetic information and found that raising HDL levels may not make any difference to heart disease risk. The study claims that individuals who inherit genes that give them naturally higher HDL levels throughout their lives have no lower an incidence of heart disease than those who inherit slightly lower levels, and is therefore skeptical of the benefits of foods or medications that will increase this type of cholesterol. I don't believe that we should throw out the HDL theory that it is an important risk factor for heart and vascular disease, but instead, we need to start looking more closely at it, including the subclasses of HDL. There is a specific HDL subclass (HDL2b) that is directly involved in removing cholesterol from the blood and preventing plaque buildup. The more of your HDL carried in this subclass, the more efficient your body is at removing cholesterol and preventing plaque buildup. Routine bloodwork doesn't single out subclasses: I believe that physicians and patients need to add more detailed tests to their routine screening. Berkeley HeartLabs and Cleveland Heartlab are leaders in this field.

- **Stress tests can determine your risk for heart attacks:** Stress tests detect arteries that are more than 70 percent blocked. However, 86 percent of heart attacks occur from arteries that are less than 70 percent blocked. It is fairly common for people to pass a stress test and then die from a heart attack a short time later. It's far more important to know if there is plaque in the artery and if it is stable or vulnerable. Coronary artery calcium scores and carotid ultrasound studies provide this information. See recommended testing at the end of the chapter for the best preventive medical approach for identifying early plaque buildup.

■ **We are all the same:** Conventional medicine treats all men the same when in fact we are all very different—all unique. We have different genetic makeups, which means that there is no such thing as a "one-size-fits-all medical protocol" to optimum health. Some of us are aspirin-sensitive and can reduce our risk of a heart attack by taking a baby aspirin every day, while others are resistant to aspirin therapy and won't benefit by taking it. There are multiple other genetic variants that inhibit otherwise effective drugs such as Plavix and certain proton pump inhibitors. It's essential that physicians recognize which genotype their patients have before prescribing these drugs. Unfortunately, this is rarely the case. The more we know about our genetic makeup the more information our health-care providers will be able to use in determining best care options. Genetic testing is available through Berkeley Labs and is performed on blood samples.

For Heart Disease, Prevention Is Key

An exercise program combined with the right nutritional therapy—the Life Plan—can reverse heart disease. It also improves heart function, reduces several coronary risk factors, enhances psychosocial well-being after a heart attack, and improves long-term survival. Both resistance training and cardiovascular workouts strengthen the heart muscle. Regular exercise reduces total cholesterol and triglyceride levels, raises HDL (good) cholesterol, and lowers LDL (bad). Aerobic exercise and resistance training can help reduce blood pressure. Many men who adhere to a regular, specifically prescribed aerobic exercise program like mine can reduce their blood pressure without taking drugs—avoiding potentially toxic side effects and the considerable expense of long-term drug therapy. Finally, exercise can also restore physical function following a stroke—a benefit not shared by drugs or surgery.

Diabetes is intrinsically linked to heart disease; in fact, elevated fasting insulin level (hyperinsulinemia) may be the most powerful predictor of heart disease. Constant surges of blood sugar and insulin not only make you fat, they increase your blood pressure. However, as you follow the Life Plan and your body fat disappears, your insulin resistance diminishes, reducing all of the inflammatory proteins that cause vascular disease leading to stroke and heart attack.

But sometimes lifestyle changes just aren't enough. Talk to your doctor about the following preventive strategy that I use with my patients. It might save your life:

- Assess your risk with the right testing.

- Find disease.

- Treat symptoms as well as the cause of the symptoms.

HEART HEALTH TERMS YOU SHOULD KNOW

Atherosclerosis: The thickening of the artery wall as a result of the accumulation of fatty material such as cholesterol, which leads to the formation of plaque. Atherosclerosis is a chronic disease that typically goes unnoticed for decades.

CIMT: Carotid intima-media thickness. This is a measurement of the thickness of the lining of the carotid artery in your neck. It is a valuable tool for physicians in clarifying cardiovascular risk and monitoring the atherosclerotic process.

Plaque: The collection of excess cholesterol that is deposited over many years in the artery walls. Plaque can be soft or hard (calcified). Hard, calcified plaque is stable and not nearly as dangerous as soft plaque, which is considered both unstable and vulnerable. Soft plaque is made up of inflammatory proteins that can cause it to break apart and enter the bloodstream. If this happens, a blood clot instantly forms on the injured site, and the flow of blood can be blocked, causing a heart attack or stroke.

Triglycerides: The fat that is found in body fat tissue. Excess triglycerides are linked to coronary artery disease, diabetes, inflammation, cancer, and Alzheimer's disease.

THINK YOU MAY HAVE HEART DISEASE?

There are easy ways to know what's going on in the vascular system without succumbing to open-heart surgery:

- Dental X-rays—calcified arteries

- Extremity X-rays—calcified arteries

- CXR—calcified arteries

- Abdominal X-rays—calcified arteries

- Cerebral images—calcified arteries

- Carotid duplex—stenosis; plaque

- Retinal scanning—atherosclerotic lesions

   Your doctor can also assess the health of the endothelium by ordering these tests:

- **Serum Markers**
  - Endothelin (ET-1)
  - Interleukin-6 (IL-6)
  - Tumor necrosis factor (TNF)
  - C-reactive protein (CRP)

- **Cellular Markers**
  - Endothelial progenitor cells (cep Cs)

- **Physiological measurement**

- **Flow-mediated dilation of the brachial artery**
  - Peripheral arterial tonometry (PAT)
  - A/B Index

Sexual Fitness

- -

Although the public is vastly more educated about erectile dysfunction, or ED, thanks to ubiquitous ads, many men are still embarrassed by the subject and hesitant to talk to their doctors. Let me assure you that there's nothing to be embarrassed about. Your doctor can help you restore your sex life to a level any man would be proud of. But you have to take the first step, and your doctor needs to take the time to talk with you. What's more, it's critical that you do address the issue, because aside from the problem of living with a disappointing sex life, your sexual function is actually a window into your total health. Your ability to maintain an erection and achieve orgasm on an average of three times a week is a key benchmark that you're healthy and physically fit. If you're not keeping up, you may be out of shape in more ways than you thought.

First, you should also know that you are not alone. Erectile dysfunction, which is defined as the persistent inability to attain or maintain an erection, affects over 30 million American men, an estimated 34 percent of men ages 40 to 70.

SIGNS OF SEXUAL HEALTH DECLINE

- Body image interferes with your confidence.

- Ejaculations become less forceful.

- Libido wanes.

- More time or stimulation for arousal is necessary.

- Orgasms may be shorter and less intense.

ED Is More than You Think

ED continues to be perceived by physicians, patients, and third-party payers (the insurance industry) as a quality-of-life issue. The truth is, ED is also an important signal that you may be suffering from heart problems. As I mentioned in the last chapter, ED is directly associated with cardiovascular disease, hypertension, diabetes, and Metabolic Syndrome. In fact, one of the first signs of heart disease is a reduction in penile hardness. An August 2010 study in the *Journal of Sexual Medicine* showed that typically, men have ED issues four to five years before their first heart attack. That's why I assume ED is a vascular disease that can lead to a heart attack or stroke—until proven otherwise.

Erectile dysfunction is directly connected to another type of "ED," this time concerning the endothelium, which is associated with circulation. Endothelial dysfunction can be the first rung of the atherosclerosis ladder, leading to heart disease and stroke. The penis is actually composed of an extensive endothelial surface interlaced with smooth muscle. Atherosclerosis (plaque buildup in your arteries) can occur throughout the body. So if the arteries supplying your heart with blood have atherosclerosis—or heart disease—it's not surprising that the smaller arteries of your penis are affected. For that matter, because of their size, the arteries of the penis may narrow sooner than the arteries in your heart. This is exactly why ED is an early warning sign for heart disease and may be a predictive sign of stroke later in life.

Many "silent" disease processes can also affect the endothelium, which can then cause a decrease in erectile function. These can include:

- Diabetes

- Hyperlipidemia

- Hypertension

- Hypogonadism

- Metabolic Syndrome

- Neurological diseases

- Neurological trauma

- Obesity

- Parkinson's disease

- Testosterone deficiency

Risk Factors That Signal ED-Related Cardiovascular Disease

Almost 90 percent of men with ED have at least one risk factor for heart disease. If you have any of the following, take this book to your doctor so that you can have a thoughtful conversation not just about ED but about heart disease, and then get the proper testing.

Age: Men under 50 experiencing ED are at high risk that their sexual dysfunction is linked to heart disease.

Weight: Obesity is a strong predictor of heart disease and has an associated higher risk of ED.

Diabetes: Narrows and hardens penile blood vessels, which increases a diabetic's odds for ED.

Cholesterol levels: Men with elevated LDL (bad cholesterol) are twice as likely to have ED.

High blood pressure: Hypertension clinics frequently report a high prevalence of ED. In fact, two out of three men with hypertension notice changes in their erectile function.

Hormonal imbalances: A common denominator in most of these medical conditions is testosterone deficiency—which is linked to a higher degree of atherosclerotic obstruction and greater heart disease risk, not to mention ED.

Lifestyle—smoking/drinking: These are independent risk factors for ED that are also associated with atherosclerosis. Smoking, like alcohol, can impair blood vessel health.

Medications: Blood pressure medications, along with antidepressants (such as Prozac, Paxil, and Zoloft), acid-blockers, and even antihistamines, can all affect performance and desire.

The Truth about ED Prescription Drugs

It is possible to reverse erectile dysfunction and improve your sex life. Often, the first line of defense for many physicians is medication. In the standard-issue 10-minute office visit you'll probably be handed a prescription for Viagra®, Cialis®, or Levitra®. Instead of instantly asking for medication, I recommend that you take with you a copy of the Sexual Health Inventory for Men (SHIM), a wonderful tool that can help spark a frank and clear conversation with your physician. The form is available at www.njurology.com/_forms/shim.pdf. Then, talk to your doctor about your problem, and be as specific as possible.

ED drugs are classified as PDE-5 inhibitors, and include the brand names Viagra, Levitra, and Cialis. They are all designed to improve endothelial function and, subsequently, to correct ED issues. These drugs may well improve endothelial function everywhere, including the blood vessels going to the heart and brain. I believe there's a good chance that in the future these drugs will be approved for the treatment of heart disease and used for stopping the progression of vascular disease, heart attack, and stroke.

Yet these erectile-enhancing drugs aren't magic in a bottle, no matter what you may have heard from your friends. They're not going to help plummeting hormone levels or elevated blood sugar levels. And these drugs can have a negative impact on your whole body. Like many medications, they can produce side effects such as dangerous drops in blood pressure, hearing loss, vision difficulties, and the much-talked-about four-hour erection. Research findings published in the May 2010 *Archives of Otolaryngology—Head and Neck Surgery* showed that men over 40 who were taking oral erectile dysfunction drugs had doubled their risk for hearing loss.

Before you start popping prescription pills, work with the Life Plan to take off a few pounds. A 2003 Harvard study linked men with BMIs greater than 28 with more than a 30 percent higher risk of ED than men whose BMIs were less than 23. In fact, 80 percent of men with moderate to severe erection problems are overweight or obese. By focusing on low-fat/low-glycemic nutrition, the right exercise, nutraceuticals, and hormone correction (when/if clinically indicated), you can prevent, delay, and even reverse sexual health issues.

Exercise Improves Sexual Fitness

If you're looking for just one more reason to get to the gym, think of this: Men who are sedentary are much more likely to have ED than men who are physically active. This is because passionate sex requires higher levels of physical fitness. In fact, sex is a form of exertion that can be harmful to men with advanced heart disease.

Let me put this as bluntly as possible: The harder you work out the better your erections will be. The latest research suggests that improving muscle strength/tone, endurance, body composition, and cardiovascular function are key to a prolonged sex life. Exercise boosts you psychologically, reduces stress, increases confidence, and elevates your mood.

Every aspect of the Life Plan workouts is necessary. You may find it surprising, but the most important component of sexual fitness is flexibility. Unfortunately, it's also the component that is most ignored. But as you embrace your Pilates workouts, you'll find that you literally begin to loosen up. Sex will become much more comfortable, and you might be able to explore new sexual positions that you just weren't able to get yourself into before.

The resistance training is important because it naturally raises your testosterone levels, which, as you've learned, are important for optimum sexual function. Cardio will help melt the pounds away so you'll feel better about the way you look in bed, and frankly, that's often half the battle.

Men often kid around with me about specific strength-training exercises they can do to tone up their penis, but there really is an answer. I tell all my patients, even those without sexual function issues, that they need to work Kegel exercises into their daily strength-training routine. These exercises strengthen the pubococcygeus muscle (PC), and can make erections stronger and harder and improve ejaculatory control.

The first step is to isolate your PC muscle. The next time you have to urinate, stop your flow midstream. The muscles you use to do that are part of the PC. But don't make this a habit, because interrupting urine flow can cause bladder issues. Then, when you are not urinating, contract this muscle 10 times in a row, and then increase your reps to 20–30 as you get stronger. You can also consult *The Life Plan* for more variations on this exercise if it gets too boring. It will take three to four weeks before you notice a difference, but keep at it. The results are worth the wait.

Good Sex Comes from a Good Night's Sleep

Poor sleep has been linked with ED, especially if you suffer from obstructive sleep apnea syndrome (OSAS). Sleep apnea disrupts the stage of sleep in which you experience rapid eye movement (REM), and this is when erections while sleeping normally occur. The REM disruption results in fewer erections, which affects your overall sexual health. It is also believed that inflammation plays a strong part in sexual dysfunction, because CRP (C-reactive protein), a solid indicator of inflammation, is increased in patients diagnosed with OSAS.

Sleep apnea is directly linked to the obesity epidemic. If you have been told that you snore loudly, wake up in the middle of the night gasping for air, or feel constantly fatigued in the morning, you may have OSAS. The best way to find out is to discuss this with your doctor and participate in a sleep study, which will confirm your suspicions. The most common treatment involves sleep with a device called a C-PAP, which, while not that sexy, will definitely keep you alive and ultimately can help improve your sex life.

Getting a good night's sleep can actually improve many aspects of your health. A 2010 study published in the journal *Sleep* determined that seven hours is the minimum magic number of hours asleep that you should be trying to achieve. Anything less can increase risk of developing cardiovascular disease. What's more, a recent Mayo Clinic study further linked sleep deprivation to obesity. The study found that people who achieved less than five hours of sleep a night consumed 549 additional calories during the day. In another study, published in 2012 in the *Journal of Clinical Endocrinology & Metabolism*, it was shown that a poor night's sleep can activate the appetite-controlling part of the brain, increasing levels of hunger throughout the day.

TESTOSTERONE AND ENDOTHELIAL HEALTH

Low testosterone is another predictor of atherosclerosis. Interestingly, men with established coronary heart disease display reduced circulating testosterone levels, which are often associated with a certain degree of erectile dysfunction independently of other vascular risk factors. This suggests a protective role of testosterone in the endothelium.

Sometimes, It Is Just in Your Head

Erectile dysfunction is not the only problem that men face in the bedroom. Some men complain that they have just lost their libido: their sexual desire and creativity. Others have issues with discomfort or timing, as they either take too long to ejaculate or orgasm too quickly. These issues may be more emotional than physical. I can tell you that often, issues with sex can be resolved when you change the way you think about sex and your relationships.

I created the following tables for a recent speaking engagement on male sexual health based on an article I read in *Men's Health* magazine. It shows me that the average American man is looking for, and getting, less than average sexual activity. Sex is not just a barometer of your health, it's also a much-needed release (literally) from the stresses of everyday life, and a crucial way to share a loving bond with your partner. See how you compare with the following to determine how your current level of sexual activity ranks with the rest of the world. If you fall into the category of "average American," I can tell you right now that you need to do better. Then, follow my lead so that you can have more active, passionate sex. Just as you have learned to get your body into better shape, you can also master the emotional side of sexual fitness.

NUMBER OF TIMES PER WEEK THE AVERAGE MAN HAS SEX:

1. Korea   4.5
2. Greece   4.2
3. Romania   4.0
4. Philippines   3.9
5. Russia   3.8

   United States   **2.9**

   World Average   2.8

AVERAGE DURATION OF SEX (IN MINUTES), FROM FOREPLAY TO CLIMAX:

1. Mexico   23.1
2. Netherlands   22.4
3. Spain   22.3
4. Brazil   21.8
5. France   21.7

   United States   **17.7**

   World Average   19.16

AVERAGE NUMBER OF SEXUAL POSITIONS IN THE AVERAGE MAN'S ARSENAL:

1. Hungary   8.2
2. Argentina   5.7
3. Spain   4.6

4.	Brazil	3.9
5.	Greece	3.8
	United States	**2.7**
	World average	3.3

PERCENTAGE OF MEN WHO HAVE TAKEN A PERFORMANCE-ENHANCING PILL:

1.	**United States**	**21.0%**
2.	South Africa	14.9%
3.	United Kingdom	14.7%
4.	Netherlands	12.8%
5.	Philippines	12.5%
	World Average	11.0%

Tips for Increasing Sexual Fitness

- -

Keep the lines of communication open: Talk about your health issues with both your doctor and your spouse or partner. Being honest about all aspects of your life, particularly your health, your stress levels, and what you desire sexually, is the doorway to true intimacy. Talk about what feels great and what does not for yourself as well as your partner.

Think of new options: Explore ways to incorporate a more fulfilling sexual life into your day, especially if you have health issues that are holding you back from experiencing the full range of sexual activity. Focus on contact, touching, kissing, playful caressing throughout the day. Shake up your routine, from the days and times you usually have sex to new positions. Fuel the romance with special "dates" and, above all, keep a positive outlook with your mate. As your body begins to change and you have more energy, you may quickly see that your sexual desire returns.

Focus on your partner: I've met hundreds of men over the years who approach sex as a sport, and they're always the ones who want to be first to the finish line. I have two words of advice for these guys: SLOW DOWN. If you can begin to be more present during sex instead of wondering how long you could go or how fast you can perform, you'll find that you—and your partner—can experience even more pleasure from it.

Sarcopenia

THINK YOU MAY HAVE ED? TALK TO YOUR DOCTOR ABOUT THESE DIAGNOSTICS

- DEXA scan for body composition

- Lab tests: C-reactive protein, testosterone/free testosterone, estradiol, DHT, LH, lipid panel, HgA1c, homocysteine

- Specialized testing: EndoPat 2000 (the leading medical device for noninvasive endothelial function)

As we age, the most dramatic and significant decline that we can outwardly notice is in our lean body mass and strength. These two ultimately determine every aspect of our quality of life, including sex: Overall weakness leads to sexual dysfunction. Together, they are known as sarcopenia, which is further defined by having an 18 percent or greater loss of lean body mass when compared to younger men in their twenties.

Sarcopenia occurs as muscle mass is slowly replaced by body fat. You may notice that you can't lift heavy objects as easily as you did before, even if you aren't dropping weight. Unfortunately, most men don't reduce their caloric intake as they age, causing body fat to gradually increase each year as they lose muscle tissue. For example, the average 25-year-old man has 20 percent body fat, but by 55 that jumps to 30 percent and by 75 it's 35 percent. It typically begins in your early forties, progressing at 3 to 5 percent for that decade and increasing to 10 or 20 percent per decade after age 50. The average man can expect to gain roughly one pound of fat every year between the ages of 30 and 60, while losing about a half pound of muscle mass each year. And from age 60 on it gets even worse. The largest loss of muscle mass occurs between ages 50 and 75, with a total average loss of 25 percent.

The problem is that it affects not only the way you look but the way you feel and how fast you age. The pounds you gain are making you look older and out of shape, and affect every other aspect of your health. Without muscle you cannot produce the correct levels of both growth hormone and testosterone. At the same time, poor muscle mass increases the production of the hormone cortisol, which not only makes you feel anxious, but also adds to your growing waistline in the form of additional belly fat. Because it takes more effort to exercise when you have weak muscles, you may put it off entirely, leading to increased physical inactivity and further deconditioning.

At the same time, the loss of muscle mass makes you look and feel weak because you *are* getting weaker. From age 60 onward, your energy levels will decline and frailty ensues, affecting your bones and your ability to move around. As you start losing bone mass, your muscle mass also declines. According to the National Osteoporosis Foundation, two million men have osteoporosis and another 12 million are at risk, yet osteoporosis in men remains "underdiagnosed and underreported." In my practice, there isn't a week that goes by that I don't see a male patient who is osteopenic (the start of osteoporosis), osteoporotic, or sarcopenic—sometimes all three. The good news is that all of these disorders can be turned around with comprehensive diagnostics, correcting hormone deficiencies, the right nutrient supplementation (calcium, vitamin D3), and weight-bearing exercise (resistance training).

WHAT CAUSES SARCOPENIA?

- Diminished protein metabolism
- Decline in natural hormone levels
- Spinal cord changes
- Decline in physical activity
- Poor nutrition
- Cellular dysfunction

Muscle and strength loss can be stopped and reversed only with resistance exercise. Balance and coordination also improve with weight-lifting, which reduces our chance of falling—a major source of injury, fractures, and debilitation, leading to death for men as they age.

Avoiding frailty is critical because it is the number-one reason for nursing home admissions. Sadly, most doctors are not addressing it correctly. Frailty can be easily assessed by undergoing a DEXA scan, which measures body composition and bone density.

The Life Plan Can Help Resolve Illness

It's very obvious that losing weight can reverse many diseases, including diabetes, heart disease, and obesity. But dropping pounds is not enough to fight sarcopenia and other devastating illnesses that make you feel old. These require a more physically fit body, and the only way to accomplish that is through exercise. A 2002 study published in the *New England Journal of Medicine* concluded that exercise capacity is perhaps the most powerful predictor of life span. Exercise has also proven to be an effective strategy for preventing or reversing a host of other diseases:

- **Arthritis.** Men with rheumatoid or degenerative arthritis benefit from exercise, which improves endurance, strengthens muscles, and increases both joint flexibility and range of motion. These benefits can't be realized with drugs or surgery.

- **Cancer.** Evidence suggests physical activity reduces the risk for colon cancer.

- **Chronic obstructive pulmonary disease (COPD).** Adding exercise to a COPD rehabilitation program can result in both physiological and psychological benefits, even for those with severe air flow obstruction or asthma.

- **Depression.** Aerobic exercises such as walking and running reduce depression and anxiety, improve stress tolerance, enhance self-image, and increase one's sense of well-being. Plus, exercise stimulates the release of your own "feel good" hormones (endorphins).

- **Diabetes.** Exercise can prevent, delay, or even reverse the serious complications of diabetes, namely, vascular disease of the brain, heart, kidneys, eyes, and legs.

- **Osteoporosis.** High-intensity strength training will prevent and actually reverse bone loss and other degenerative bone diseases.

Finding the Right Doctor

So when should you start your health action plan? Now and not a minute later. The first step is to find a doctor whom you can work with. Unfortunately, that's not always easy. I believe that men who are looking to proactively take care of their health deserve more than just 10-minute office visits. We deserve detailed and continuing counseling on how to manage aging and prevent disease.

Taking this book to your doctor along with any checklists or quizzes you completed from the book is an excellent way of clearly demonstrating what your health goals are, and how you want to proceed in accomplishing them. If you bring this book to your doctor and he or she points to my picture and tells you that you will NEVER look like this, it's time to look for another doctor. There is no reason you cannot reverse disease and get your body into the best shape of your life. Anyone who tells you differently is simply not fully informed about healthy aging, which is what this program is all about. And who would want to be treated by someone who can't manage your health as you age, or who is not using all the knowledge and tools available?

For example, in my office we offer every patient a comprehensive health evaluation that begins with a complete physical exam and intensive set of diagnostics that are used to establish baseline health records. These tests reveal your weakest health links and your health strengths. We also provide an exercise assessment and nutrition consultation so that every patient leaves my office with a clear understanding of what he needs to do in terms of diet and exercise to improve his health. I also perform a full-body composition test using DEXA scanning, as well as strength testing and a comprehensive cognitive assessment. These are all standard issue for healthy aging practices, and you should be receiving the same from your doctor.

Whether or not you are in the market for a new physician, here is a list of what I consider the most important questions you need to ask your doctor regarding your health and medical care. These 10 questions will be your medical shopping list that you need to have answered before you start the program. If you don't like the answers you receive, it may be time to find yourself a new doctor.

1. If costs and insurance were not an issue, what would you do to improve my quality of life and reduce my risks for age-related disease?

2. What nutritional supplementation do you recommend that will reduce my risks for disease and possibly extend my life span?

3. What are your thoughts about correcting hormonal deficiencies?

4. Do HMOs or insurance companies affect or influence your decisions on what medications, diagnostic tests, or referrals to specialists you make regarding my medical care?

5. If you or a member of your family had my condition, what would you do?

6. When you refer me to a specialist, would this be the same person you would use if *you* had this same problem?

7. Is your compensation affected by your prescribing patterns, referral patterns, or the diagnostic tests you order?

8. How do you feel about government or insurance guidelines regarding screening?

9. What role do you believe diet and exercise have in your practice? How much training have you had in the role nutrition and exercise play in healthy aging?

10. Do you practice what you preach?

Tests Every Man Must Request

We also have the right to know our current health status each and every year, which can be done completely only by proactively screening for silent diseases. Today, many of the following tests are discouraged by insurance carriers that state that these medical tests are "unnecessary." This must change. Request that you receive these tests as frequently as noted, and some testing may need to be performed by a specialist. You may need to talk with your insurance carrier to determine if they are covered. If they aren't, see if you can work with your doctor to assess the costs before the testing.

ASSESS YOUR HEALTH AT HOME

Review this list before you see your doctor. None of these are signs of healthy aging: All are signs of potential diseases that can—and should—be eliminated or reversed. Make sure your doctor understands that these conditions are not acceptable, no matter what your age:

- Belly fat
- Bone loss/osteoporosis
- Constant fatigue
- Depression
- Diabetes
- Erectile dysfunction
- Flabby muscles
- Gain of 10 pounds or more over past year or two
- High LDL score
- Increased joint stiffness
- Irritability/emotional swings/anxiety
- Lethargy midmorning or midafternoon
- Loss of libido
- Loss of muscle/loss of strength
- Poor skin quality, reduced elasticity
- Reduced flexibility
- Reduced work productivity
- Sleep disturbances
- Trouble concentrating/slow recall/foggy thinking

Test	Definition	Optimal Results
DEXA Scan for Bone Density and Body Composition	This fast, painless, noninvasive procedure determines whether you are at risk for osteoporosis, which causes bones to become fragile or break. A DEXA scan can be used to monitor osteoporosis treatment as well as compute body composition (body fat percentage and muscle weight). DEXA is not the same as a bone scan, which detects fractures, cancer, infections, and other abnormalities. Men over 45 should complete a DEXA scan annually. This is typically performed in physicians' offices that own these machines. Some doctors may send you to a diagnostic center for these studies.	Percent body fat <15% T Score >= 0
Blood Pressure	Blood pressure is the force exerted by circulation blood on the walls of blood vessels and is one of the principal vital signs. Maximum blood pressure is called systolic and minimum is diastolic. It is typically measured in millimeters of mercury. This test is performed in your doctor's office and should be done at least annually as well as during any sick visit.	120/80 or less

CANCER SCREENINGS

Test	Definition	Optimal Results
Colonoscopy	This test provides an inside look at your colon and rectum. Preparation for the test and the test itself are painless. If polyps (possible precancerous growths) are detected they can be easily removed. This procedure is handled by a gastroenterologist and is recommended for men starting at age 50 and should be repeated every 5 to 10 years. Men with a family history of polyps or colon cancers should consult their health professional to determine when to start and how often they should repeat their colonoscopies.	Negative
Digital Rectal Exam of the Prostate	Used to screen overall prostate health. This exam should be performed every year in your doctor's office during a typical physical. It is recommended that African-American men and any man with a family history of prostate cancer begin having annual digital rectal exams at the age of 40. Caucasian men should start at age 45.	Negative
Prostate Specific Antigen (PSA)	This blood test is used to screen for prostate cancer before symptoms occur and should be performed at least once a year. If the level increases the test needs to be repeated in 2–3 weeks, and if still elevated, patient needs to see a urologist.	0–3 ng/mL

BLOOD SUGAR CONTROL

Test	Definition	Optimal Results
Hemoglobin A1c (Glycohemoglobin)	This blood test provides a long-term look at blood sugar control. This test should be taken 2–3 times a year.	< 5.5%

Test	Definition	Optimal Results
Insulin (Fasting)	This blood test provides information about your body's sensitivity to insulin. Elevated levels can indicate insulin resistance, a major cause of Type 2 diabetes. This is typically performed 2–3 times a year.	< 5 uIU/mL
Glucose (Fasting)	A blood glucose test measures the amount of glucose (sugar) in the blood. This is typically performed 2–3 times a year.	65–95 mg/dL
OGTT (Oral Glucose Tolerance Test)	A 1-hour and 2-hour glucose tolerance test can detect insulin resistance and new-onset diabetes. This can be taken in the doctor's office once or twice a year.	2hrs < 140mg/dl

CARDIAC

Test	Definition	Optimal Results
CIMT (Carotid Intima-Media Thickness)	This test consists of an ultrasound that assesses vascular age and can predict heart attack and stroke because it measures atherosclerosis and plaque character. It is considered "the mammogram of cardiovascular disease" because of its safety and accuracy. This is typically performed once a year.	Negative
ABI (Ankle-Brachial Index)	A simple test that compares the blood pressure in your arm with the blood pressure in your ankle. Test detects peripheral artery disease and predicts cardiovascular mortality. This can be performed in the doctor's office annually.	> 0.90
AAA Screen (Abdominal Aortic Aneurysm Screen)	An ultrasound of the abdominal aorta to detect aneurysms and atherosclerosis. Recommended for men 50–69 years old with at least one cardiovascular risk factor or African-Americans and all men 70 years old or older. This is typically performed annually.	Negative
Cardiac Stress Testing	This test evaluates blood flow and determines if there are blockages interfering with the supply of blood and oxygen to your heart. It also provides valuable information regarding the fitness of your heart, blood vessels, and lungs. The test is performed on a treadmill or bike, while EKG, heart rate, blood pressure, and oxygen levels are monitored and recorded. This test can be completed in a clinic or hospital. Men age 45 and over should perform this test on an annual basis.	Negative

CARDIAC BLOOD TESTS

Test	Definition	Optimal Results
Homocysteine	High homocysteine levels can injure blood vessel walls and are indicators of your risk for heart disease, Alzheimer's disease, stroke, and vascular disease. These levels should be checked annually.	< 9 umol/L

Test	Definition	Optimal Results
C-Reactive Protein (CRP)	This blood test measures silent inflammation and is used to assess risk for cardiovascular disease and all age-related diseases. CRP is typically tested at the same time a cholesterol screening is performed and is recommended as part of an annual blood chemistry screening.	<1.0 mg/l
Lipoprotein (a)-C [Lp (a)-C]	This test provides additional information about your risk of developing heart disease. It is not included in routine blood work but should be performed annually. This test is beneficial for men with existing vascular disease or who have a strong family history of coronary artery disease.	0–30 mg/dL
LDL	LDL (bad cholesterol) is obtained as part of your annual cholesterol panel and is also used to predict your risk of heart attack or stroke. This test should include LDL particle size. Small particles cause plaque buildup to progress much faster.	< 70 mg/dL
HDL and HDL Subclass-HDL2b (Berkeley Labs)	HDL (good cholesterol) is obtained as part of your annual cholesterol panel. Low levels of HDL2b put you at increased risk for heart disease.	> 50 mg/dL
Triglycerides	Triglycerides are measured along with cholesterol as part of an annual routine lipid panel test. Elevated triglyceride levels put you at risk for heart disease.	< 100 mg/dL
ApoB	A blood test that is the single most significant and consistent lipid measurement to predict heart disease risk. The test should be performed annually.	< 100 mg/dL
GFR (Glomerular Filtration Rate)	A blood test that assesses kidney function. It is a predictor of cardiovascular risk. The test should be performed annually.	> 60
F_2-isoprostanes	An annual blood test that predicts risk of coronary artery disease. F2-IsoPs are the "gold standard" for measuring oxidative stress.	< 0.86 ng/mg
Vitamin D, 25-OH	An annual blood test that identifies a Vitamin D deficiency.	50mg–100/dL
"The PLAC test" LpPLA2 (PLAC 2)	The PLAC Test predicts risk for a stroke and heart disease. Should be performed annually.	< 180
Microalbumin/Creatine Ratio (MACR)	A simple and inexpensive urine test that is excellent for predicting cardiovascular disease risk and early diabetic kidney disease. Can be performed annually.	< 4.0µg/mg
Fibrinogen	A blood test that is a sensitive indicator of inflammation and risk for heart disease. Should be performed annually.	< 450
Myeloperoxidase (MPO)	A blood test that is a strong indicator of a heart attack. Should be performed annually.	< 480 pmol/L
NT-pro BNP	Powerful test for cardiac dysfunction—the "heart happy" test. Should be performed annually.	< 125 pg/mL

Test	Definition	Optimal Results

GENETIC TESTING: These tests need to be performed only once to determine if you are at risk for various diseases. Some are essential for guiding drug therapy.

Test	Definition	Optimal Results
CYP2C19 Genotype	Helps predict response to Plavix. Should be performed on anyone considering Plavix therapy.	Results vary depending on genotype
TCF7L2	Genetic risk test for Type 2 diabetes.	Negative
APO E Genotype	Genetic test used to guide dietary and statin therapy for people who are at risk for heart disease.	Results vary depending on genotype
KIF6	Genetic test that is a valuable predictor of risk for heart disease and value of statin therapy.	Results vary depending on genotype
LPA-Aspirin Genotype	Predicts risk for heart disease and value of aspirin therapy.	Results vary depending on genotype
9p21Genotype	Predicts early-onset heart attacks and abdominal aortic aneurysms (AAA).	Results vary depending on genotype

HORMONES

Test	Definition	Optimal Results
Thyroid Panel	Thyroid hormones are analyzed through a blood sample to determine if symptoms such as fatigue, depression, cold intolerance, hair loss, headaches, fluid retention, unexplained weight gain or loss, anxiety, and panic attacks are caused by thyroid abnormalities. As needed.	
Thyroid Stimulating Hormone (TSH)	TSH screening is used to diagnose and monitor treatment of thyroid disorders. TSH levels help determine if you have hypothyroidism (production below normal) or hyperthyroidism (production above normal). As needed.	0.4–2.0 mu/L
Free T3	Used to help diagnose thyroid abnormalities. As needed.	300–420 pg/dL
Free T4	Used to help diagnose thyroid abnormalities. As needed.	0.8–1.8 ng/dL
Total Testosterone	This blood test is used to measure the total amount of testosterone in the bloodstream. Can be performed annually unless you are being treated with testosterone replacement therapy. Then every 3 to 4 months.	700–1100 ng/dL
Free Testosterone	Free testosterone is the amount of unbound testosterone found in the blood. Can be performed annually or every 3 to 4 months if you are on replacement therapy.	130–210 pg/mL 0.4–2.0 mu/L
Dihydrotesterone (DHT)	Elevated DHT levels can cause hair loss and prostate enlargement. It is a breakdown product of testosterone metabolism. As needed.	25–75 ng/dL
Estradiol, High-Sensitivity	Men who are on testosterone replacement therapy should have their estradiol levels checked every 3–6 months.	10–40 pg/mL

Test	Definition	Optimal Results
ADRENAL		
Dehydroepiandrosterone (DHEA)	A blood test to determine low DHEA levels that are correlated to symptoms including depression, obesity, lupus, Alzheimer's disease, loss of bone density, cardiovascular disease, and chronic fatigue syndrome. As needed.	350–500 mcg/dL
Cortisol (Morning Level)	This blood test is used to measure the total amount of cortisol (stress hormone) in the bloodstream. Can be performed annually.	< 18 mcg/dL
PITUITARY		
Insulin-like Growth Factor-1, Somatomedin-C, IGF-1 (indirect assay of growth hormone)	IGF-1 levels are directly related to growth hormone secretion from the pituitary gland. Can be performed annually.	200–320 ng/mL

GET YOUR EYES AND HEARING CHECKED

You should also have these complete exams every two to four years if you are between 40 and 65. Make sure your eye doctor provides glaucoma testing to make sure the pressure in your eyes is not elevated and an Amsler grid test to evaluate central vision and rule out macular degeneration.

Important Information about Prostate Specific Antigen (PSA) Screening

This test had been previously recommended for men starting at age 45, or men age 40 if there is a family history of prostate cancer or if they are of African-American heritage. A recent recommendation has changed this. The U.S. Preventative Services Task Force is a panel made up of primary care doctors, the same M.D.s who made the unpopular recommendation that mammograms were unnecessary for women under 50. In 2012 the USPSTF changed its position on the benefits of PSA screening from inconclusive to NO BENEFIT to men less than 75 years of age. They believe that early PSA screening has led to overdiagnosis and overtreatment, and that screening was associated with false positives leading to unnecessary biopsies. They extended their recommendation to high-risk groups, including African-American males and those with a family history of prostate cancer.

I do not agree with these findings, and neither do many specialists. PSA has led to a decrease in deaths from prostate cancer, a drop of 38 percent in the last 20 years. The American Urological Association believes that these findings did not adequately reflect the benefits of PSA testing and that this recommendation was "inappropriate and irresponsible." For example, Dr. H. Ballentine Carter, director of urology at Brady Urological Institute at Johns Hopkins, believes that PSA is the only screening test that we currently have that saves lives when used correctly. He recommends that physicians review PSA history in each individual and make decisions based on changes. This is why I continue to use PSA testing as an important tool for diagnosing early prostate cancer. It has proved to be a valuable part of my diagnostic evaluation of all my male patients.

ASK DR. LIFE

NAME: **Rob S.**

QUESTION: **Hello, Dr. Life, I think your book is awesome ! I'm a 41-year-old male with a testosterone level of 500. Do you think that number is way too low? Am I a D- student? Any info would be great!**

ANSWER: **The normal range for total testosterone is between 300 and 1,000 nanograms per deciliter. Levels between 200 and 300 ng/dl are considered borderline; levels below 200 ng/dl indicate a clear deficiency. If your test comes back with a testosterone level in the 100–200 range, a traditional doctor may say that you're in the normal range. For my patients, I suggest that they stay in the upper normal range, meaning that I'm looking for them to have testosterone levels of 900, 1,000, or even 1,100. Your level of 500 isn't bad and you probably don't need replacement therapy. You can increase this significantly, however, with the right kind of exercise and nutrition/supplementation, which I have discussed in previous chapters.**

• • •

Once you have a clear understanding of your current health, you can master the Life Plan, knowing that you are taking care of yourself the best way possible.

CHAPTER 11

Getting Better Every Year

I'm grateful for so many of the wonderful things that have happened since I published *The Life Plan*. The fan mail I've received and the media attention have been overwhelming at times. I'm proud of the many men who have written to let me know how their lives have changed for the better by following my program. I even received a couple of letters from women, thanking me for helping their men get back into life, in every way imaginable.

But honestly, the person I'm most proud of is . . . me. When I went to do my photo shoot to create the pictures in this book, my photographer, Terry Goodlad, told me that I looked even better than I did when he shot the images for the first book, when I was 72! I knew that I had pretty much stayed in good shape, but to

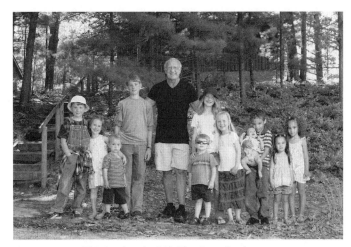

This is what the Life Plan is really about—
spending time with all of my grandkids!

hear it from a photographer who works with supermodels and professional athletes really got me thinking. And as I reviewed what has happened over the past few years I realized that even though I did get older, I got better. My body is leaner, more defined, and healthier than ever before. My heart disease still continues to reverse, and I hope that one day I'll have a completely clean bill of health. Meanwhile, I'm still riding my motorcycle, and I'm still practicing martial arts. I'm traveling to be with my grandkids, all 11 of them. I just moved into a new home with my wife, and I'm seeing patients and giving medical lectures to other doctors who are literally half my age.

The same can be true for every man who reads this book, including you. You have the power to improve so that you can continue to do the things you love today and for years to come. Just by reading this book you've taken the first steps to change. You now have all the tools necessary to enhance every aspect of your health, from internal disease to external appearance.

As you've learned from many of my patients interviewed for this book, the first few weeks will be challenging. But as you keep at it, you'll master whatever it is that you are looking for: better health, great sex, or a stronger, leaner body. So keep going, stop moaning, and stay on the program for however long it takes to reach your goals.

If you need more words of encouragement, remember the following lesson that Terry, my friend and photographer, has taught me. Whenever I have to work harder in the gym, or pass up my favorite slice of cake everyone else is enjoying, I think of what he has told me:

"Do you see anything you'd like to change in that mirror? You have the power, the ability, and the opportunity. I've met so many men who see what they need to do but can only ache for what was lost. You can change the world, by changing yourself . . . and all you have to do is take control. Truly great men mark history by taking the pain, swallowing the fear, facing their demons, and creating change. They learn to do what's Right. You've been given the sword, the greatest sword, and you will be the great warrior you are destined to be."

Acknowledgments

This book would not have been possible without the love and support of my wife, Annie. I consider myself incredibly fortunate that she entered my life when she did, and she continues to provide me with the incentives I need to achieve optimal health. And a special thanks for all the great recipes she has provided for my book.

I would also like to acknowledge my agent, Carol Mann, and all the folks at Atria Books. Sarah Durand and Judith Curr continue to support my vision, and their entire team has been tremendous to work with. My publicist, Sandi Mendelson, has been a huge resource in helping get my message out to men.

My writer, Pam Liflander, is not only a great person but a truly gifted writer who was able to help me get all my thoughts and beliefs on paper, and

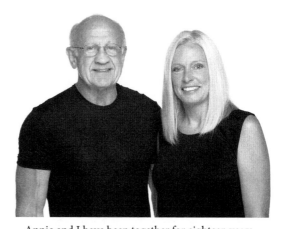

Annie and I have been together for eighteen years.

then organize and craft them into words that perfectly describe what men need to know to stay healthy and avoid feeling old.

I also want to thank the many people who have been integral to my success and the success of my books. Rod Stanley, my trainer and friend, has helped me reach a whole new level of fitness and physique; he also helped me craft and improve the exercise and nutrition chapters. Lauren Tancredi has played a huge role keeping me on task and sharing her honest opinions.

Terry Goodlad, my photographer, motivator, and dear friend, did a fantastic job encouraging me and capturing me at my very best. I'd also like to thank the folks at One Queensridge Place, Las Vegas, Nevada, who graciously allowed us to shoot the instructional photographs in their space. Joey Carson, executive producer and owner of Ex Nihilo, is a truly amazing videographer. I thank him for putting together incredible footage of what I do, and for his friendship.

Shane Gagne, my Pilates instructor, has turned a stiff old guy into a flexible, youthful guy and contributed substantially to the description of my Pilates exercises. John Adams and the entire Cenegenics Team continue to play a pivotal role in my professional success. Without Cenegenics I would never have been able to share my story. And last, but certainly not least, Dr. Phil, for supporting me and the Life Plan.

References

1. The Life Plan Philosophy

Mozaffarian, Dariush, M.D., Dr.P.H., Hao, Tao, M.P.H., Rimm, Eric B., Sc.D., Willett, Walter C., M.D., Dr.P.H., and Hu, Frank B., M.D., Ph.D. Changes in diet and lifestyle and long-term weight gain in women and men. *N. Engl. J. Med.* 2011, 364:2392–2404.

2. The Life Plan Diets

Blatt, A. D., Roe, L. S., and Rolls, B. J. Hidden vegetables: an effective strategy to reduce energy intake and increase vegetable intake in adults. *Am. J. Clin. Nutr.* 2011, Feb., ajcn.009332.

3. My Favorite Foods

Ackard, D. M., Kearney-Cooke, A., and Peterson, C. B. Effect of body image and self-image on women's sexual behaviors. *International Journal of Eating Disorders.* 422–429. Article first published online: 2000, Oct. 23, | DOI: 10.1002/1098-108X(200012)28:4<422::AID-EAT10>3.0.CO;2-1.

Golan, R., Schwarzfuchs, D., Stampfer, M. J., and Shai, I. Halo effect of a weight-loss trial on spouses: the DIRECT-Spouse study. *Public Health Nutrition.* 2010, 13:544–549.

4. Supplementing the Life Plan Diets

Nissen, S., Sharp, R., Ray, M., Rathmacher, J. A., Rice, D., Fuller, J. C., Jr., Connelly, A. S., and Abumrad, N. Effect of leucine metabolite beta-hydroxy-beta-methylbutyrate on muscle metabolism during resistance-exercise training. *Journal of Applied Physiology.* 1996, Nov., 2095–2104.

9. Hormone Optimization: The Absolute Truth

Albert, S. Low-dose recombinant human growth hormone as adjuvant therapy to lifestyle modifications in the management of obesity. *J. Clin. Endocrinol. Metab.* 2004, Feb., Vol. 89, No. 2.

American Association of Clinical Endocrinologist Medical Guidelines for Clinical Practice for Growth Hormone Use in Growth Hormone Deficient Adults and Transition Patients—October 2009 Update. *Endocrine Practice.* 2009:15(2); 1.

Annewieke, W. van den Beld, de Jong, F. H., et al. Measures of bioavailable serum testosterone and estradiol and their relationships with muscle strength, bone density, and body composition in elderly men. *J. Clin. Endocrinol. Metab.* 2000, Vol. 85, No. 9, 3276–82.

Araujo, A. et al. Endogenous Testosterone and Mortality in Men: A Systematic Review and Meta-Analysis. *J. Clin Endocrin & Metabol.* 2011, 96(10):3007–3019.

Asbell, S. O., Raimane, K. C., Montesano, A. T., Zeitzer, K. L., Asbell, M. D., and Vijayakumar, S. Prostate-specific antigen and androgens in African-American and white normal subjects and prostate cancer patients. *J. Natl. Med. Assoc.* 2000, Sep., 92(9):445–49.

Baker, H. W., et al. Arginine-infusion test for growth-hormone secretion. *Lancet.* 1970, 2(7684):1193.

Basaria, S., Wahlstrom, J. T., and Dobs, A. S. Anabolic-androgenic steroid therapy in the treatment of chronic diseases. *J. Clin. Endocrinol. Metab.* 2001, Vol. 86, No. 11, 5108–17.

Beauregard, C., et al. Growth hormone decreases visceral fat and improves cardiovascular risk markers in women with hypopituitarism: A randomized, placebo-controlled study. *J. Clin. Endocrinol. Metab.* First published ahead of print, 2008, Apr. 1, as doi:10.1210/jc.2007-2371.

Bengtsson, B.-Å., et al. Treatment of adults with growth hormone deficiency: Results of a 13-month placebo controlled cross over study. *Clin. Endocrinol.* (Oxf.)1993, 76:309–17.

Besson, A., et al. Reduced Longevity in Untreated Patients with isolated Growth Hormone Deficiency. *J Clin Endocrin. Metab.* 2003, 88(8):3664.

Biller, B. Sensitivity and specificity of six tests for the diagnosis of adult GH deficiency. *J. Clin. Endocrinol. Metab.* 2002, May, 87(5):2067–79.

Bjorntorp, P. "Portal" adipose tissue as a generator of risk factors for cardiovascular disease and diabetes. *Arteriosclerosis.* 1990, 10:493–96.

Bohannon, R. W. Comfortable and maximum walking speed of adults aged 20–79 years: Reference values and determinants. *Age Ageing.* 1997, 26:15–19.

Bonert, V. S. Body mass index determines evoked growth hormone (GH) responsiveness in normal healthy male subjects: Diagnostic caveat for adult GH deficiency. *J. Clin. Endocrinol. Metab.* 2004, July, 89(7):3397–401.

Boquete, H. R. Evaluation of diagnostic accuracy of insulin-like growth factor (IGF)-I and IGF-binding protein-3 in growth hormone-deficient children and adults using ROC plot analysis. *J. Clin. Endocrinol. Metab.* 2003, Oct., 88(10):4702–8.

Bross, R., Javanbakht, M., and Bhasin, S. Anabolic interventions for aging-associated sarcopenia. *J. Clin. Endocrinol. Metab.* 1999, Vol. 84, No. 10, 3420–30.

Bülow, B., Hacrmar, L., Mikoczy, Z., Nordström, C. H., and Erfurth, E. M. Increased cerebrovascular mortality in patients with hypopituitarism. *Clinical Endocrinology.* 1997, 46, 75–81.

Caminiti, G., Volterrani, M., et al. Effect of long-acting testosterone treatment on function exercise capacity, skeletal muscle performance, insulin resistance, and baroreflex sensitivity in elderly patients with chronic heart failure: A double-blind, placebo controlled, randomized study. *J. Am. Coll. Cardiol.* 2009, 54:919–27.

Capaldo, B., Patti, L., Oliverio, U., Longobardi, S., Pardo, F., Vitali, F., Fazio, S., di Reller, F., Bindi, B., Lombardi, G., and Sacca, L. Increased arterial intimi-media thickness in childhood onset growth hormone deficiency. *J. Clin. Endocrinol. Metab.* 1997, 82, 1378–81.

Cappola, A. Insulin-like growth factor I and interleukin-6 contribute synergistically to disability and mortality in older women. *J. Clin. Endocrinol. Metab.* 2003, May, 88(5):2019–25.

Carani, C., Zini, D., Baldini, A., et al. Effects of androgen treatment in impotent men with normal and low levels of free testosterone. *Arch. Sex. Behav.* 1990, June, 19(3):223–34.

Carroll, P. U. et al. Growth hormone deficiency in adulthood and the effects of growth hormone replacement: A review. Growth Hormone Research Society Scientific Committee. *J. Clin. Endocrinol. Metab.* 1998, Feb., 83(2):382–95.

Carter, H. B., et al. Longitudinal evaluation of serum androgen levels in men with and without prostate cancer. *Prostate.* 1995, July, 27(1):25–31.

Cauter, E., et al. Age-related changes in slow wave sleep and REM sleep and relationship with growth hormone and cortisol levels in healthy men. *JAMA.* 2000, Aug. 16, 284, No. 7, 861–67.

Christa, C. Van Bunderen, et al. The association of serum insulin-like growth factor-I with mortality, cardiovascular disease, and cancer in the elderly: A population-based study. *J. Clin. Endocrinol. Metab.* 2010 (95) 9, 4449–54.

Chute, G. Sex hormones and coronary artery disease. *Am. J. Med.* 1987, Nov., 83(5):85359.

Cittadini, A., et al. Growth hormone deficiency in patients with chronic heart failure and beneficial effects of its correction. *J. Clin. Endocrinol. Metab.* 2009 (94), 3329–36.

Clasey, J. L., et al. Abdominal visceral fat and fasting insulin are important predictors of 24-hr GH release independent of age, gender, and other physiological factors. *J. Clin. Endocrinol. Metab.* 2001, 86(8):3845–52.

Clemmons, D. R., and Underwood, L. E. Nutritional regulation of IGF-1-1 and IGF-1 binding proteins. *Annu. Rev. Nutr.* 1991, 11:393–412.

Colao, A., Cerbone, G., Pivonello, R., Aimaretti, G., Loche, S., Di Somma, C., Faggiano, A., Corneli, G., Ghigo, E., and Lombardi, G. The growth hormone (GH) response to the arginine plus GH-releasing hormone test is correlated to the severity of lipid profile abnormalities in adult patients with GH deficiency. *J. Clin. Endocrinol. Metab.* 1999, Apr., 84(4):1277–82.

Colao, A., et al. Growth hormone treatment on atherosclerosis: Results of a 5-year open, prospective, controlled study in male patients with severe growth hormone deficiency. *J. Clin. Endocrinol. Metab.* 2008 (93)9, 3416–24.

Colao, A., Di Somma, C., Spiezia, S., Rota, F., Pivonello, R., Savastano, S., and Lombardi, G. The natural history of partial growth hormone deficiency in adults: A prospective study on cardiovascular risk and atherosclerosis. *J. Clin. Endocrinol. Metab.* 2006, June, 91(6):2191–2200.

Colao, A., et al. Short-term effects of growth hormone (GH) treatment or deprivation on cardiovascular risk parameters and intima-media thickness at carotid arteries in patients with severe GH deficiency. *J. Clin. Endocrinol. Metab.* 2005 (90)4, 2056–62.

Consensus statement. Consensus guidelines for the diagnosis and treatment of adults with GH deficiency II: A statement of the GH Research Society in association with the European Society for Pediatric Endocrinology, Lawson Wilkins Society, European Society of Endocrinology, Japan Endocrine Society, and Endocrine Society of Australia. *European Journal of Endocrinology.* 2007, 157:695–700.

Conti, E., et al. Insulin-like growth factor-1 as a vascular protective factor. *Circulation.* 2004, 110:2260–65.

Conway, H. J. Randomized clinical trial of testosterone replacement therapy in hypogonadal men. *Int. J. Androl.* 1988, Aug., 11(4):247–64.

Cooper, C. S., Perry, P. J., Sparks, A., et al. Effect of exogenous testosterone on prostate volume, serum and semen prostate specific antigen levels in healthy young men. *J. Urol.* 1998, Feb., 159(2):441–43.

Critical evaluation of the safety of recombinant human growth hormone administration: Statement from the Growth Hormone Research Society. *J. Clin. Endocrinol. Metab.* 2001, 86:1868-70.

de Boer, H., et al. Clinical aspects of growth hormone deficiency in adults. *Endocr. Rev.* 1995, 16:63–86.

Denti, L., et al. Insulin-like growth factor 1 as a predictor of ischemic stroke outcome in the elderly. *Am. J. Med.* 2004 Sep. 1, 117(5):312–17.

Doyl, G., et al. Insulin-like growth factor-3 and binding protein-3 induces early induces early apoptosis in malignant prostate cancer cells and inhibits tumor formation in vitro. *Prostate.* 2000, 5 (2):141–182.

Drake, W. M. Optimizing growth hormone therapy in adults and children. *Endocr. Rev.* 2001, Aug. 1, 22(4):425–50.

Ebert, T., Jockenhovel, F., Morales, A., et al. The current status of therapy for symptomatic late-onset hypogonadism with transdermal testosterone gel. *Eur. Urol.* 2005, Feb., 47(2):137–46.

English, K. M., Mandour, O., Steeds, R. P., Diver, M. J., Jones, T. H., and Channer, K. S. Men with coronary artery disease have lower levels of androgens than men with normal coronary angiograms. *Eur. Heart J.* 2000, June, 21(11):890–94.

English, K. M., Steeds, R. P., Jones, T. H., Diver, M. J., Channer, K. S. Low-dose transdermal testosterone therapy improves angina threshold in men with chronic stable angina: A randomized, double-blind, placebo-controlled study. *Circulation.* 2000, Oct. 17, 102(16):1906–11.

Evaluation and treatment of AGHD: An Endocrine Society clinical practice guideline. *J. Clin. Endocrinol. Metab.* 2006, 91:1621–34.

Fazio, S., et al. Effects of growth hormone on exercise capacity and cardiopulmonary performance in patients with chronic heart failure *J. Clin. Endocrinol. Metab.* 2007 (92), 11, 4218–23.

Felsing, N. E., et al. Effect of low snf high intensity exercise on circulating growth hormone in men. *J. Clin. Endocrinol. Metab.* 1992, 75(1):157–62.

Fowelin, J., Attrall, S., Lager, I., Bengtsson, B.-Å. Effects of treatment with recombinant human growth hormone on insulin sensitivity and glucose metabolism in adults with growth hormone deficiency. *Metabolism.* 1993, 42, 1443–47.

Franco, C. Growth hormone treatment reduces abdominal visceral fat in postmenopausal women with abdominal obesity: A 12-month placebo-controlled trial. *J. Clin. Endocrinol. Metab.* 2005, Mar. 1, 90(3):1466–74.

Frederick, C. W., Wu, et al. Identification of late-onset hypogonadism in middle-aged and elderly men. *N. Engl. J. Med.* 2010 (363):123–35.

Friedrick, N., et al. Mortality and Serum Insulin-Like Growth Factor (IGF)-I and IGF Binding Protein 3 Concentrations. *J. Clin. Endocrin. Metab.* 2009, 94 (5):1732–1736.

Fuhrman, B., et al. Basal growth hormone concentrations in blood and the risk for prostate cancer: a case-control study. *Prostate.* 2005 Jul 1; 64(2):109–115.

Gelato, M. Aging and immune function: A possible role for growth hormone. *Hormone Research.* 1996, 45:46–49.

Gillett, M. J., Martins, R. N., Clarnette, R. M., Chubb, S. A., Bruce, D. G., and Yeap, B. B. Relationship between testosterone, sex hormone binding globulin and plasma amyloid beta peptide 40 in older men with subjective memory loss or dementia. *J. Alzheimers Dis.* 2003, Aug., 5(4):267–69.

Giustina, A., and Veldhuis, J. D. Pathophysiology of the neuroregulation of growth hormone secretion in experimental animals and the human. *Endocrin. Rev.* 1998, 19(6):717–97.

Gouras, G. K., Xu, H., Gross, R. S., et al. Testosterone reduces neuronal secretion of Alzheimer's β-amyloid peptides. *Proc. Natl. Acad. Sci. USA.* 2000, 97:1202–5.

Hak, E. et al. Low Levels of Endogenous Androgens Increase the Risk of Atherosclerosis in Elderly Men: The Rotterdam Study. *J. Clin Endocrin & Metabol.* 2002, 87(8):3632–3639.

Hartman, M., et al. Growth hormone replacement therapy in adults with growth hormone deficiency improves maximal oxygen consumption independently of dosing regimen or physical activity. *J. Clin. Endocrin. Metab.* 2008, 93:125–30.

Hartman M. L., et al. Which patients do not require a GH stimulation test for the diagnosis of adult GH deficiency? *J. Clin. Endocrinol. Metab.* 2002, Feb., 87(2):477–85.

Hartman, M. L. Physiological regulators of growth hormone secretion. In Juul, A., and Jorgensen, J. O. L. (eds). *Growth Hormone in Adults*, 2d. ed. Cambridge: Cambridge University Press 2000, pp. 3–53.

Hoeck, H. C. Diagnosis of growth hormone (GH) deficiency in adults with hypothalamic-pituitary disorders: Comparison of test results using pyridostigmine plus GH-releasing hormone (GHRH), clonidine plus GHRH, and insulin-induced hypoglycemia as GH secretagogues. *J. Clin. Endocrinol. Metab.* 2000, Apr., 85(4):1467–72.

Hoeck, H. C. Test of growth hormone secretion in adults: Poor reproducibility of the insulin tolerance test. *Eur. J. Endocrinol.* 1995, Sep. 1, 133(3):305–12.

Hoffman, M. A., DeWolf, W. C., and Morgentaler, A. Is low serum free testosterone a marker for high grade prostate cancer? *J. Urol.* 2000, Mar., 163(3):824–27.

Hogervorst, E., Bandelow, S., Combrinck, M., and Smith, A. D. Low free testosterone is an independent risk factor for Alzheimer's disease. 2004, Nov.–Dec., 39(11–12):1633–39.

Hogervorst, E., Combrinck, M., et al. Testosterone and gonadotropin levels in men with dementia. *Neuro. Endocrinol. Lett.* 2003, 24(3–4):203–8.

Holt, R. Growth hormone: A potential treatment option in diabetes? *Diabetic Voice.* July 2003, Vol. 48. Issue 2.

http://www.ghresearchsociety.org/bin/Default.asp.

Hyde, Z., et al. Low free testosterone predicts frailty in older men: The Health in Men study. *J. Clin. Endocrinol. Metab.* 2001, Apr. 21 (95)7, 3165–72.

Jain, J. Urol effect of exogenous testosterone on prostate volume, serum and semen prostate specific antigen levels in healthy young men. *J. Urol.* 1998, Feb., 159(2):441–43.

Jankowska, E. A., Biel, B., Majda, J., et al. Anabolic deficiency in men with chronic heart failure: Prevalence and detrimental impact on survival. *Circulation.* 2006, 114:1829–37.

Johannsson, G. Growth hormone treatment of abdominally obese men reduces abdominal fat mass, improves glucose and lipoprotein metabolism, and reduces diastolic blood pressure. *J. Clin. Endocrinol. Metab.* Vol. 82, No. 3, 727–34.

Johansson, J.-Q., Landin, K., Tengboru, L., Rosén, T., and Bengtsson, B.-Å. High fibrinogen and plasminogen activator inhibitor activity in growth hormone deficient adults. *Arterioscler. Thromb.* 1994, 14:434–37.

Juul, A., et al. Low serum insulin-like growth factor-1 is associated with increased risk of ischemic heart disease: A population-based case-control study. *Circulation.* 2002, 106:939–44.

Juul, A. Serum levels of insulin-like growth factor I and its binding proteins in health and disease. *Growth Horm. IGF-1 Res.* 2003, 13:113–70.

Kapoor, D., Malkin, C. J., Channer, K. S., et al. Androgens, insulin resistance and vascular disease in men. *Clin. Endocrinol.* (Oxf). 2005, 63:239–50.

Khaw, K. T., and Barrett-Connor, E. Blood pressure and endogenous testosterone in men: An inverse relationship. *J. Hypertens.* 1988, Apr., 6(4):329–32.

Khaw, K. T., and Barrett-Connor, E. Lower endogenous androgens predict central adiposity in men. *Ann. Epidemiol.* 1992, Sep., 2(5):675–82.

Khaw, K. T., Dowsett, M., Folkerd, E., et al. Endogenous testosterone and mortality due to all causes, cardiovascular disease, and cancer in men: European prospective investigation into cancer in Norfolk (EPIC-Norfolk). Prospective Population Study. *Circulation.* 2007, 116:2694–2701.

Khosla, S., Melton, L. J., III, and Elizabeth, J. Relationship of serum sex steroid levels and bone turnover markers with bone mineral density in men and women: A key role for bioavailable estrogen. *J. Clin. Endocrinol. Metab.* 1998, Vol. 83, No. 7, 2266–74.

Kwan, A., and Hartman, M. IGF-1-1 measurements in the diagnosis of adult growth hormone deficiency. *Pituitary.* 2007, 10(2):151–57.

Kwan, M., Greenleaf, W. J., Mann, J., Crapo, L., and Davidson, J. M. The nature of androgen action on male sexuality: A combined laboratory self-report study on hypogonadal men. *J. Clin. Endocrinol. Metab.* 1983, Vol. 57, 557–62.

Larsen, Kronnenberg, Melmed, and Polonsky (eds). *Williams Textbook of Endocrinology.* Saunders, 2003, 10th ed. Chapter 8, authored by Shlomo Melmed and David Kleinberg, summarizes Adult Somatotropin Deficiency in Table 8-20, p. 226, and they point out that IGF-1 levels may be "low or normal" in adult deficiency states.

Larsson, S. C., et al. Association of diet with serum insulin-like growth factor I in middle-aged and elderly men. *Am. J. Clin. Nutr.* 2005, 81:1163–67.

Laughlin, G., et al. Low Serum Testosterone and Mortality in Older Men. *J. Clin Endocrin & Metabol.* 2008, 93(1):68–75.

Laughlin, G., et al. The prospective association of serum insulin-like growth factor I (IGF-I) and IGF-binding protein-1 levels with all cause and cardiovascular disease mortality in older adults: the Rancho Bernardo Study. *J. Clin. Endocrinol. Metab.* 2004, Jan. 1, 89(1):114–20.

Le Corvoisier, P., et al. Cardiac effects of growth hormone treatment in chronic heart failure: A meta-analysis. *J. Clin. Endocrinol. Metab.* 2007 (92)1, 180–85.

Liu, J., Tsang, S., and Wong, T. M. Testosterone is required for delayed cardioprotection and enhanced heat shock protein 70 expression induced by preconditioning. *Endocrinology.* 2006, 147:4569–77.

Maggio, M. et al. Relationship Between Low Levels of Anabolic Hormones and 6-Year Mortality in Older Men. *Arch. Intern. Med.* 2007, 167(20):2240–2254.

Makimura, H., et al. Reduced growth hormone secretion is associated with increased carotid intima-media thickness in obesity. *J. Clin. Endocrinol. Metab.* 2009 (94) 12, 5131–38.

Malkin, C. J., et al. Testosterone therapy in men with moderate severity heart failure: A double-blind randomized placebo controlled trial. *European Heart Journal.* 2006, 24, 54–64.

Malkin, C. J., Pugh, P. J., Jones, R. D., et al. The effect of testosterone replacement on endogenous inflammatory cytokines and lipid profiles in hypogonadal men. *J. Clin. Endocrinol. Metab.* 2004, 89:3313–18.

Marcello, Maggio, et al. Relationship between low levels of anabolic hormones and 6-year mortality rate in older men. *Archives of Internal Medicine.* 2007 (167), 20, 2249–54.

Margolese, H. C. The male menopause and mood: Testosterone decline and depression in the aging male—is there a link? *J. Geriatr. Psychiatry Neurol.* 2000, Summer, 13(2):93–101.

Marin, P., Holmang, S., Jonsson, L., Sjostrom, L., Kvist, H., et al. The effects of testosterone treatment on body composition and metabolism in middle-aged obese men. *Intl. J. Obes. Relat. Metab. Disord.* 1992, Dec., 16(12):991–97.

Marin, P., Krotkiewski, M., and Bjorntorp, P. Androgen treatment of middle-aged, obese men: Effects on metabolism, muscle and adipose tissues. *Eur. J. Med.* 1992, Oct., 1(6):329–36.

Markussis, V., Beshyah, S. A., Fischer, C., Sharp, P., Nicolaides, A. N., and Johnson, D. G. Detection of premature atherosclerosis by high resolution ultrasonography in symptom-free hypopituitary adults. *Lancet.* 1992, 340, 1188–92.

Meinhardt, U., M.D., et al. The effects of growth hormone on body composition and physical performance in recreational athletes: A randomized trial. *Annals of Internal Medicine.* 2010, May 4 (152), 9, 568–77.

Melmed, S. Supplemental growth hormone in healthy adults: The endocrinologist's responsibility. *Nature Clinical Practice.* 2006, 2:119.

Menke, A., et al. Sex steroid hormone concentrations and risk of death in US men. *American Journal of Epidemiology.* 2009 (171) 5, 583–92.

Moffat, S. D., et al. Free testosterone and risk for Alzheimer disease in older men. *Neurology.* 2004, Jan. 27, 62(2):188–93.

Morley, J. E. Testosterone replacement and the physiologic aspects of aging in men. *Mayo Clin. Proc.* 2000, Jan., 75 Suppl:S83–87.

Movérare-Skrtic, S., et al. Serum insulin-like growth factor-I concentration is associated with leukocyte telomere length in a population-based cohort of elderly men. *J. Clin. Endocrinol. Metab.* 2009, Dec. (94), 12, 5078–84.

Mukherjee, A. Seeking the optimal target range for insulin-like growth factor I during the treatment of adult growth hormone disorders. *J. Clin. Endocrinol. Metab.* 2003, Dec., 88(12):5865–70.

Muller, M., Grobbee, D. E., den Tonkelaar, I., Lamberts, S. W., and van der Schouw, Y. T. Endogenous sex hormones and metabolic syndrome in aging men. *J. Clin. Endocrinol. Metab.* 2005, May, 90(5):2618–23.

Muller, M. Endogenous sex hormones and cardiovascular disease in men. *J. Clin. Endocrin. Metab.* 2003, Vol. 88, No. 11, 5076–86.

Murray, R., Bidlingmaier, M., Strasburger, C., and Shalet, S. The diagnosis of partial growth hormone deficiency in adults with a putative insult to the hypothalamo-pituitary axis. *J. Clin. Endocrinol. Metab.* 2007, 92(5):1705–9.

Murray, R. D., Adams, J. E., and Shalet, S. M. Adults with partial growth hormone deficiency have an adverse body composition. *J. Clin. Endocrinol. Metab.* Apr., 89(4):1586–91.

Murray, R. D., and Shalet, S. M. Insulin sensitivity is impaired in adults with varying degrees of GH deficiency. *J. Clin. Endocrinol.* 2005, Feb., 62(2):182–88.

O'Carroll, R., and Bancroft, J. Testosterone therapy for low sexual interest and erectile dysfunction in men: A controlled study. *Br. J. Psychiatry.* 1984, Aug., 145:146–51.

O'Connor. Ph.D. Thesis, Dublin, 1998.

Ohlsson, C. et al. High Serum Testosterone is Associated with Reduced Risk of Cardiovascular Events in Elderly Men. The MrOS (Osteoporotic Fractures in Men) Study in Sweeden. *J. Am. Coll. Cardiol.* 2011, 58(16):1674–1684.

Pandian, R., and Nakamoto, J. M. Rational use of the laboratory for childhood and adult growth hormone deficiency. *Clin. Lab. Med.* 2004, Mar., 24(1):141–74.

Paoletti, A. M., et al. Low androgenization index in elderly women and elderly men with Alzheimer's disease. *Neurology.* 2004, Jan. 27, 62(2):301–3.

Papasozomenos, S. Ch., and Shanavas, A. Testosterone prevents the heat shock-induced overactivation of glycogen synthase kinase-3 beta but not of cyclin-dependent kinase 5 and c-Jun NH2-terminal kinase and concomitantly abolishes hyperphosphorylation of tau: implications for Alzheimer's disease. *Proc. Natl. Acad. Sci. USA.* 2002, Feb. 5., 99(3):1140–45.

Pasarica, M., et al. Effect of growth hormone on body composition and visceral adiposity in middle-aged men with visceral obesity. *J. Clin. Endocrin. Metab.* 2007, 92:4265–70.

Popovic, V., et al. Serum insulin-like growth factor I (IGF-I), IGF-binding proteins 2 and 3 and the risk for development of malignancies in adults with growth hormone (GH) deficiency treated with GH: Data from KIMS (Pfizer International Metabolic Database). *J. Clin. Endocrinol. Metab.* 2010 (online).

Pugh, P., Jones, T. H., and Channer, K. Acute haemodynamic effects of testosterone in men with chronic heart failure. *European Heart Journal.* 2003, 24, 909–15.

Ramzi, R. H., Kaiser, F. E., and Morley, J. E. Outcomes of long-term testosterone replacement in older hypogonadal males: A retrospective analysis. *J. Clin. Endocrinol. Metab.* 1997, Vol. 82, No. 11, 3793–96.

Rasmussen, M. H., et al. Massive weight loss restores 24-hr growth hormone release profiles and serum insulin-like growth factor-1 levels in obese subjects. *J. Clin. Endocrinol. Metab.* 1995, 80(4):1407–15.

Rhoden, E. L., and Morgentaler, A. Risks of testosterone-replacement therapy and recommendations for monitoring, *N. Engl. J. Med.* 2004, Jan. 29, 350(5):482–92.

Rosén, T., and Bengtsson, B.-Å. Premature mortality due to cardiovascular disease in hypopituitarism. *Lancet.* 1990, 336, 285–88.

Rosenfeld, R. G., Cohen, P., Robison, L. L., Bercu, B. B., Clayton, P., Hoffman, A. R., Radovick, S., Saenger, P., Savage, M. O., and Wit, J. M. Long-term surveillance of growth hormone therapy. *J. Clin. Endocrinol. Metab.* 2012, Jan., 97(1):68–72. Epub 2011, Dec. 15.

Roubenof, R. Cytokines, insulin-like growth factor-1, sarcopenia, and mortality in very old community-dwelling men and women: The Framingham Heart Study. *Am. J. Med.* 2003, Oct. 15, 115(6):429–35.

Rupprecht, R. Neuroactive steroids: Mechanisms of action and neuropsychopharmacological properties. *Psychoneuroendocrinology.* 2003, Feb., 28(2):139–68.

Sattler, F. R., et al. Testosterone and growth hormone improve body composition and muscle performance in older men. *J. Clin. Endocrinol. Metab.* 2009 (94) 6, 1991–2001.

Savastano, S., et al. Growth hormone treatment prevents loss of lean mass after bariatric surgery in morbidly obese patients: Results of a pilot, open, prospective randomized controlled study. *J. Clin. Endocrinol. Metab.* 2009 (94), 3, 817–26.

Savine, R., and Sonksen, P. Growth hormone-hormone replacement for somatopause. *Horm. Res.* 2000, 53 (Suppl. 3): 37–41.

Shalender, B., and Tenover, J. S. *Age-Associated Sarcopenia—Issues in the Use of Testosterone as an Anabolic Agent in Older Men. J. Clin. Endocrinol. Metab.* 1997, Vol. 82, No. 6, 1659–60.

Shores, M. M., Matsumoto, A. M., Sloan, K. L., et al. Low serum testosterone and mortality in male veterans. *Arch. Intern. Med.* 2006, 166:1660–65.

Shores, M. M., Smith, N. L., Forsberg, C. W., Anawal, B. D., and Matsumoto, A. M. Testosterone treatment and mortality in men with low testosterone levels. *J. Clin. Endocrinol. Metab.* 2012, 97:2050–58.

Simpson, H., et al. Growth hormone replacement therapy for adults: Into the new millennium. *Growth Horm. IGF Res.* 2002, 12:1–33.

Skakkebaek, N. E., Bancroft, J., Davidson, D. W, and Warner, P. Androgen replacement with oral testosterone undecenoate in hypogonadal men: A double blind controlled study. *Clin. Endocrinol.* (Oxf). 1981, 14:49–61.

Skeleton, D. A., et al. Strength, power & related functional ability of healthy people aged 60–89 years. *Aging People.* 1994, 23:371–77.

Snel, Y. E., et al. Magnetic resonance image-assessed adipose tissue and serum lipid and insulin concentrations in growth hormone deficient adults: Effects of growth hormone replacement. *Arterioscler. Thromb. Vasc. Biol.* 1995, 15:1543–48.

Snyder, P., Peachey, H., Hannoush, P., et al. Effect of testosterone treatment on bone mineral density in men over 65 years of age. *J. Clin. Endocrinol. Metab.* 1999, Vol. 84, No. 6, 1966–72.

Snyder, P. The effects of testosterone treatment on body composition and metabolism in middle-aged obese men. *Intl. J. Obes. Relat. Metab. Disord.* 1992, Dec., 16(12):991–97.

Society for Endocrinology, Practice and Policy, Growth Hormone. http://www.endocrinology.org/policy/docs/gh.html.

Srinivas-Shankar, U. Effects of testosterone on muscle strength, physical function, body composition and quality of life in intermediate-frail and frail elderly men: A randomized, double-blind, placebo-controlled study. *J. Clin. Endocrinol. Metab.* 2010 (95)2, 639–50.

Stoving, R. K., et al. Low circulating insulin-like growth factor I bioactivity in elderly men is associated with increased mortality. *J. Clin. Endocrinol. Metab.* 2008 (93), 7, 2515–22.

Tan, R. S., and Pu, S. J. A pilot study on the effects of testosterone in hypogonadal aging male patients with Alzheimer's disease. *Aging Male.* 2003, Mar., 6(1):13–17.

Tenover, J. S. Effects of testosterone supplementation in the aging male. *J. Clin. Endocrinol. Metab.* 1992, Oct., 75(4):1092–98.

Tong, P. C., Ho, C. S., Yeung, V. F., et al. Association of testosterone, insulin-like growth factor-I, and C-reactive protein with metabolic syndrome in Chinese middle-aged men with a family history of type 2 diabetes. *J. Clin. Endocrinol. Metab.* 2005, 90:6418–23.

Toogood, A. A., et al. Beyond the somatopause: Growth hormone deficiency in adults over the age of 60 years. *J. Clin. Endocrinol. Metab.* 1996, 82:460–65.

Urban, R. J., Bodenbrug, Y. H., et al. Testosterone administration to elderly men increases skeletal muscle strength and protein synthesis. *Am. J. Physiol.* 1995, Nov., 269 (5 Pt 1): E820–26.

Vahl, N., et al. Abdominal adiposity and physical fitness are major determinants of the age associated decline in stimulated GH secretion in healthy adults. *J. Clin. Endocrinol. Metab.* 1996, 81(6):2209–15.

Vahl, N., et al. Abdominal adiposity rather than age and sex predicts mass and regularity of GH secretion in healthy adults. *Am. J. Physiol.* 1997, 272:E1108–16.

Vasan, R. S., et al. Serum insulin-like growth factor-1 and risk for heart failure in elderly individuals without a previous myocardial infarction: The Framingham Heart Study. *Ann. Intern. Med.* 2003, 139:642–48.

Veldhuis, J. D. Neuroendocrine control of pulsatile growth hormone release in human: Relationship with gender. *Growth Hormone IGF-1 Res 8* (Suppl B). 1998, 49–59.

Vestergaard, P., and Hoeck, H. C. Reproducibility of growth hormone and cortisol responses to the insulin tolerance test and the short ACTH test in normal adults. *Horm. Metab. Res.* 1997, Mar., 29(3):106–10.

Webb, C. M., Adamson, D. L., de Zeigler, D., and Collins, P. Effect of acute testosterone on myocardial ischemia in men with coronary artery disease. *Am. J. Cardiol.* 1999, Feb. 1, 83(3):437–39, A9.

Weltman, A., et al. Endurance training amplifies the pulsatile release of growth hormone: Effects of training intensity. *J. Appl. Physiol.* 1992, 72(6):2188–96.

Weltman, A., et al. Relationship between age, percentage body fat, fitness and 24-hour growth hormone release in healthy young adults: Effect of gender. *J. Clin. Endocrinol. Metab.* 1994, 78:543–48.

Wu, F. C., and von Eckardstein, A. Androgens and coronary artery disease. *Endocr. Rev.* 2003, 24:183–217.

Wu, S. Z., and Weng, X. Z. Therapeutic effects of an androgenic preparation on myocardial ischemia and cardiac function in 62 elderly male coronary heart disease patients. *Chin. Med. J.* (Engl.). 1993, June, 106(6):415–18.

Yazdanpasah, M., et al. An insulin-Like Growth factor-1 Promoter Polymorphism is Associated With Increased Mortality in Subjects With Myocardial Infarction in an Elderly Caucasian Population. *Am J Cardiol.* 2006, 93:1274–1276.

Young, A. Muscle function in old age. *New Issue Neuroscience.* 1998, I:141–56.

Yuen, K., et al. Is lack of recombinant growth hormone (GH)-releasing hormone in the United States a setback or time to consider glucagon testing for adult GH deficiency? *J. Clin. Endocrin. Metab.* 2009, 94, 2702–7.

Zmuda, J. M., Cauley, J. A., Kriska, A., Glynn, N. W., Gutai, J. P., and Kuller, L. Longitudinal relation between endogenous testosterone and cardiovascular disease risk factors in middle-aged men: A 13-year follow-up of former Multiple Risk Factor Intervention Trial participants. 1997, Oct. 15, 146(8):609–17.

10. The Life Plan and Your Doctor

Akishita, M., Hashimoto, M., Ohike, Y., Ogawa, S., Iijima, K., Eto, M., et al. Low testosterone level is an independent determinant of EDys in men. *Hypertens. Res.* 2007, 30:1029–34.

Alberto, C. O. Bidirectional dopaminergic modulation of excitatory synaptic transmission in orexin neurons. *J. Neuroscience.* 2006, 26.39:10043–50.

Asahara, T., Masuda, H., Takahashi, T., Kalka, C., Pastore, C., Silver, M., et al. Bone marrow origin of endothelial progenitor cells responsible for postnatal vasculogenesis in physiological and pathological neovascularization. *Circ. Res.* 1999, 85:221–28.

Aversa, A. Drugs targeted to improve endothelial function: Clinical correlates between sexual and internal medicine. *Curr. Pharm. Des.* 2008, 14:3698–99.

Aversa, A., Rossi, F., Francomano, D., Bruzziches, R., Bertone, C., Santiemma, V., et al. Early endothelial dysfunction as a marker of vasculogenic erectile dysfunction in young habitual cannabis users. *Intl. J. Impot. Res.* 2008b, 20:566–73.

Ballard, S. A., Gingell, C. J., Tang, K., Turner, L. A., Price, M. E., and Naylor, A. M. Effects of sildenafil on the relaxation of human corpus cavernosum tissue in vitro and on the activities of cyclic nucleotide phosphodiesterase isozymes. *J. Urol.* 1998, 159:2164–71.

Beavo, J. A. Cyclic nucleotide phosphodiesterases: Functional implications of multiple isoforms. *Physiol. Rev.* 1995, 75:725–48.

Bhatt, D. L., Steg, P. G., Ohman, E. M., Hirsch, A. T., Ikeda, Y., Mas, J. L., et al. International prevalence, recognition, and treatment of cardiovascular risk factors in outpatients with atherothrombosis. *JAMA*, 2006, 295:180–89.

Billups, K. L., Bank, A. J., Padma-Nathan, H., Katz, S., and Williams, R. Erectile dysfunction is a marker for cardiovascular disease: Results of the Minority Health Institute expert advisory panel. *J. Sex. Med.* 2005, 2:40–50; discussion 50–52.

Bocchio, M., Pelliccione, F., Passaquale, G., Mihalca, R., Necozione, S., Desideri, G., et al. Inhibition of phosphodiesterase type 5 with tadalafil is associated to an improved activity of circulating angiogenic cells in men with cardiovascular risk factors and erectile dysfunction. *Atherosclerosis.* 2008, 196:313–19.

Conti, E., et al. Insulin-like growth factor-1 as a vascular protective factor. *Circulation.* 2004, 110:2260–65.

Cooke, J. P. The endothelium: A new target for therapy. *Vasc. Med.* (London). 2000, 5:49–53.

Denti, L., et al. Insulin-like growth factor 1 as a predictor of ischemic stroke outcome in the elderly. *Am. J. Med.* 2004, Sep. 1, 117(5):312–17.

Eguchi, M., Masuda, H., and Asahara, T. Endothelial progenitor cells for postnatal vasculogenesis. *Clin. Exp. Nephrol.* 2007, 11:18–25.

Feldman, H. A., Goldstein, I., Hatzichristou, D. G., Krane, R. J., and McKinlay, J. B. Impotence and its medical and psychosocial correlates: Results of the Massachusetts Male Aging Study. *J. Urol.* 1994, 151:54–61.

Forest, C., Ferlin, A., De Toni, L., Lana, A., Vinanzi, C., Galan, A., et al. Circulating endothelial progenitor cells and endothelial function after chronic Tadalafil treatment in subjects with erectile dysfunction. *Intl. J. Impot. Res.* 2006, 18:484–88.

Forest, C., Lana, A., Cabrelle, A., Ferigo, M., Caretta, N., Garolla, A., et al. PDE-5 inhibitor, vardenafil, increases circulating progenitor cells in humans. *Intl. J. Impot. Res.* 2005, 17:377–80.

Fukui, M., Kitagawa, Y., Ose, H., Hasegawa, G., Yoshikawa, T., and Nakamura, N. Role of endogenous androgen against insulin resistance and atherosclerosis in men with type 2 diabetes. *Curr. Diabetes Rev.* 2007, 3:25–31.

Goldstein, I., Lue, T. F., Padma-Nathan, H., Rosen, R. C., Steers, W. D., Wicker, P. A. Oral sildenafil in the treatment of erectile disfunction. *N. Engl. J. Med.* 1998, 338(20): 1397–1404.

Guay, A. T. ED2: Erectile dysfunction/endothelial dysfunction. *Endocrinol. Metab. Clin. North Am.* 2007, 36:453–63.

Jackson, G., Rosen, R. C., Kloner, R. A., and Kostis, J. B. The second Princeton consensus on sexual dysfunction and cardiac risk: New guidelines for sexual medicine. *J. Sex. Med.* 2006, 3:28–36; discussion 36.

Kostis, J. B., Jackson, G., Rosen, R., Barrett-Connor, E., Billups, K., Burnett, A. L., et al. Sexual dysfunction and cardiac risk (the Second Princeton Consensus Conference). *Am. J. Cardiol.* 2005, 96:85M–93M.

Lin, C. S. Phosphodiesterases as therapeutic targets. *Urology.* 2003, 61:685–91.

Masuda, H., Kalka, C., and Asahara, T. Endothelial progenitor cells for regeneration. *Hum. Cell.* 2000, 13:153–60.

McMahon, C. Comparison of efficacy, safety, and tolerability of on-demand tadalafil and daily dosed tadalafil for the treatment of erectile dysfunction. *J. Sex. Med.* 2005, 2:415–25; discussion 425–27.

McMahon, C. Efficacy and safety of daily tadalafil in men with erectile dysfunction previously unresponsive to on-demand tadalafil. *J. Sex. Med.* 2004, 1:292–300.

Montorsi, P., et al. Is erectile dysfunction the "tip of the iceberg" of a systemic vascular disorder? *European Urology* 44. 2003, 352–54.

Reffelmann, T., and Kloner, R.A. Cardiovascular effects of phosphodiesterase 5 inhibitors. *Curr. Pharm. Des.* 2006, 12:3485–94.

Rosano, G. M., Leonardo, F., Pagnotta, P., Pelliccia, F., Panina, G., and Cerquetani, E. Acute anti-ischemic effect of testosterone in men with coronary artery disease. *Circulation.* 1999, 99:1666–70.

Selvin, E., Burnett, A. L., and Platz, E. A. Prevalence and risk factors for erectile dysfunction in the US. *AMJ.* 2007, Feb.,Vol. 120, Issue 2, 151–57.

Solomon, H., Man, J. W., and Jackson, G. Erectile dysfunction and the cardiovascular patient: Endothelial dysfunction is the common denominator. *Heart.* 2003, 89:251–53.

Ther. Adv. Urol. 2009 (4):179–97.

Thompsom, I. M., Tangen, C. M., Goodman, P. J., Probstfield, J. L., Moinpour, C. M., and Coltman, C. A. Erectile dysfunction and subsequent cardiovascular disease. *JAMA.* 2005, 294:2996–3002.

Volkow, N. D., and Wise, R. A. How can drug addiction help us understand obesity? *Nature Neuroscience.* 2005, 8.5, 555–60.

Index

A

abdomen, fat around, 1, 16, 20, 75, 88, 205–6, 220, 222, 224, 228–29, 231, 257, 261

abdominal muscles:
abdominal crunch, 115, 157
ab machine, 127–28, 154
bicycle crunch, 158–59
double leg extension for abs, 105
Dr. Life's secret ab stretch, 114
exercises and, 104–5, 114–15, 119, 127–28, 154, 157–59, 165, 170
resistance band crunches, 159
single leg extension for abs, 104–5
stretches and, 104–5, 111–14, 195
supine ab series, 104
see also core/abdominal training

addictions, 238–43
breaking of, 243
food and, 238–41, 243
quizzes on, 239, 242

adductor stretch, 102, 197

African-Americans, 85, 263, 266

age, aging, 2–3, 5, 50, 90, 172, 198, 214, 237, 241, 269–70
body fat and, 204–5
diagnostic tests and, 262–64, 266
diets and, 19, 21, 23, 25, 32
doctor selection and, 259–61
exercises and, 93, 117, 119, 121, 173, 175–76, 178–79

heart disease and, 243, 250
hormones and, 219–25, 228–30, 232, 235
Life Plan philosophy and, 9–11
myths and, 12–18
sarcopenia and, 10, 15, 119, 257–58
sex and, 9, 249–50
Stanley and, 114–15
supplements and, 78–79, 85–87

alcoholic beverages, 16, 19, 29, 33, 73–74, 223, 228, 251
addictions and, 238, 242–43

almonds, 37, 41–42, 44–45, 53
Chocolate Almond Peanut Butter Shake, 70
Chocolate Almond Protein Shake, 70

Alzheimer's disease, 10–11, 247
diagnostics tests and, 263, 266
hormones and, 223, 231

amino acids, 27, 67, 71, 88–89, 233
HHD and, 40, 46–47

andropause, 9, 14, 219–20, 229

ankles, 156, 263
stretches and, 99, 107, 112–13

antioxidants, 52–53, 121
supplements and, 79–80, 82, 86–87

appetite, 11, 23, 68, 72, 74, 239, 254
journals and, 207–8
Life Plan Diets rules and, 25–26, 29–31, 33–34

arms:
barbell curl, 149
dumbbell curl, 128, 148

dumbbell overhead extension, 128, 152
exercises and, 112–13, 121, 128–37, 139–42, 147–53, 156, 158, 160–65, 169–70, 182, 211–13
EZ curl bar, 128
journals and, 205, 211–13
machine curl, 150
opposite arm leg reach, 112–13
plank opposite-arm-leg reach, 156
preacher curl, 128, 147
quadruped opposite-arm-leg reach, 158
resistance band biceps curls, 170
resistance band one-arm flies, 160
resistance band one-arm rear fly lateral raise, 164
resistance band triceps extensions, 169
stretches and, 103–5, 107, 112–13, 194
triceps pushdown, 128, 151
weighted dips, 128, 153

arthritis, 32, 78–79, 222, 259

atherosclerosis, 14, 16, 244–45
diagnostic tests and, 247–48, 263
hormones and, 224, 231, 254
sexual fitness and, 249, 251

athletes, athletics, 9, 19, 81, 87, 90, 202, 270
exercise and, 111, 115, 179–81
hormones and, 228, 230
myths and, 12–13

diets, diet (cont.)
  hormones and, 20–21, 23, 25,
    27–31, 33, 221, 227–28, 233,
    267
  journals on, 34, 90, 201–2, 207–8,
    211–13
  myths and, 14–18
  sex and, 52, 252
  of Troy, 35–36
  see also foods; Life Plan Diets;
    recipes
diet sodas, 33
digital rectal exam of the prostate,
    262
dihydrotestosterone (DHT), 257, 265
dinners, 57, 72
  BHD and, 43, 63–66
  Black Pepper Salmon with
    Asparagus Spears, 63
  FBD and, 46, 63–66
  HHD and, 49, 63–64, 66
  Not So Naked Chicken, 64
  Quinoa Tabbouleh, 64
  Tempeh Tagine, 66
  Turkey Stir-Fry, 65
disease:
  Life Plan philosophy and, 9–10
  prevention of, 3, 12–13, 21,
    79–81, 87–88, 90, 175–76, 237,
    246–47, 252, 258–59
  reversal of, 2, 4, 11–12, 229, 237,
    246, 252, 258–59, 270
DNA, 10, 54, 79, 231
docosahexanoic acid (DHA), 84
doctors, 119, 259–61
dopamine, 238–39
dyslipidemia, 119, 230

E

eccentric contraction, 124
eggs, egg whites, 37, 39, 53, 67, 201
  BHD and, 41, 59
  FBD and, 44, 59
  HHD and, 47
  Life Plan Diets rules and, 27–28
  Poached Egg with Smoked
    Salmon, 59
eicosapentaenoic acid (EPA), 84
endorphins, 176, 259
endothelium, 176, 257
  heart disease and, 16, 231, 244,
    248–49, 254

hormones and, 230–31, 254
myths and, 15–16
sexual fitness and, 249–51, 254
energy, 2, 21, 36, 68, 74, 118–19,
    121, 176, 198, 241, 256
  body fat and, 23, 204
  diets and, 20, 23, 25, 32–33, 40,
    211
  exercise and, 23, 177, 184, 199,
    213
  hormones and, 114, 221–22,
    229
  Life Plan philosophy and, 9–11
  myths and, 17–18
  supplements and, 79, 86
erectile dysfunction (ED), 14–15,
    224, 241, 248–54, 261
  diagnostic tests and, 253, 257
  exercise and, 177–78, 252
  heart associated with, 249–52
  medications for, 251–52, 256
  supplements and, 88–89
essential fatty acids (EFAs), 31,
    77–78, 82, 84, 87
estradiol, 257, 265
estrogen, 229, 235
exercises, exercise, 1, 3–4, 31–32,
    73–74, 93–173, 175–207,
    237–38, 257–60
  body fat and, 88, 117–18, 175–80,
    182–83, 185, 200
  Dave and, 198–200
  diets and, 20–23, 25, 27, 32, 34,
    97, 118, 171, 175–76, 186,
    209
  food addiction and, 241, 243
  goal setting and, 202–3
  at gym, 4, 11, 13, 17, 36, 88, 96,
    118, 126–55, 172, 209–10,
    212–15
  heart disease and, 119, 176–77,
    179–81, 244–46, 259
  at home, 118, 155–70, 210–12
  hormones and, 118, 126, 221–23,
    227–28, 231, 233, 252–53, 259
  journals and, 184, 201–2,
    211–13
  Life Plan philosophy and, 9, 11
  myths and, 12–18
  with personal trainers, 35, 90, 95,
    114, 126, 171, 182, 213–15
  protein shakes and, 67–68, 97,
    171, 186

on the road, 4, 118, 155–70,
    210–11
sarcopenia and, 15, 119, 257–58
sex and, 94, 111, 126, 177–78,
    182, 209, 252–53
supplements and, 79–81, 88–89,
    120
vacations from, 213
see also specific types of training
    and workouts
eyes, 107, 259, 266
Ezekiel bread, 31, 37, 39, 41–43,
    45, 48

F

fat, body, 11–12, 40, 67–68, 74, 119,
    214, 241
  around abdomen, 1, 16, 20, 75,
    88, 205–6, 220, 222, 224,
    228–29, 231, 257, 261
  diets and, 19–27, 29–31, 36, 50,
    117, 177
  exercise and, 88, 117–18, 175–80,
    182–83, 185, 200
  goal setting and, 202, 204
  heart disease and, 246–47
  hormones and, 177, 220–22, 224,
    228–29, 231–32
  journals on, 205–6
  measurements of, 204–6, 262
  supplements and, 85, 88–89
fat, dietary, 22, 24, 38, 59
  addictions and, 238–40
  BHD and, 26, 39–43
  cooking and, 49, 52–53
  FBD and, 43–46
  HHD and, 40, 46–49
  hormones and, 227, 233
  Life Plan Diets rules and, 26–28,
    30–31, 33
  saturated, 30, 43, 53, 68, 233
  supplements and, 28, 46, 77–78,
    82, 84, 87, 90, 120
Fat-Burning Diet (FBD), 40, 43–46,
    50, 52, 202
  food suggestions for, 44–46
  recipes and, 56–66
fatigue, 1–2, 14, 198, 240, 253, 261,
    266
  diets and, 26, 33, 35–36
  exercise and, 124, 177, 180
  hormones and, 220, 222, 230, 235